S0-AKP-260

KHBlocker MD

August 1973

SLEEP RESEARCH
AND
CLINICAL PRACTICE

Sleep Research and Clinical Practice

Edited by

GENE USDIN, M.D.

Professor of Clinical Psychiatry
Louisiana State University School of Medicine

BRUNNER/MAZEL, *Publishers* ● NEW YORK
BUTTERWORTHS ● LONDON

Copyright © 1973 by The American College of Psychiatrists
Published by BRUNNER/MAZEL, INC.
64 University Place, New York, N. Y. 10003
All rights reserved, including the right of reproduction
in whole or in part in any form.

Library of Congress Catalogue Card No. 73-79080
SBN 87630-074-3

MANUFACTURED IN THE UNITED STATES OF AMERICA

American College of Psychiatrists

Officers

1972-73

BENJAMIN BALSER, M.D., *President*
MELVIN SABSHIN, M.D., *President-Elect*
HAMILTON FORD, M.D., *First Vice-President*
HAYDEN H. DONAHUE, M.D., *Second Vice-President*
PETER A. MARTIN, M.D., *Secretary-General*
CHARLES E. SMITH, M.D., *Treasurer*
JOHN D. TRAWICK, JR., M.D., *Archivist-Historian*

Publications Committee

GENE USDIN, M.D., *Chairman*
CHARLES K. HOFLING, M.D., *Vice Chairman*

EARL BROWN, M.D.   PETER MARTIN, M.D.
PAUL J. FINK, M.D.   JOHN C. NEMIAH, M.D.
HENRY P. LAUGHLIN, M.D.   MELVIN SABSHIN, M.D.
HAROLD VISOTSKY, M.D.

CONTRIBUTORS

WILLIAM C. DEMENT, M.D.
Professor of Psychiatry, Department of Psychiatry, Stanford University School of Medicine

ANTHONY KALES, M.D.
Professor and Chairman, Department of Psychiatry, Pennsylvania State University, Milton S. Hershey Medical Center

JOYCE KALES, M.D.
Assistant Professor of Psychiatry, Department of Psychiatry, Pennsylvania State University, Milton S. Hershey Medical Center

ISMET KARACAN, M.D.
Professor of Psychiatry and Director of Sleep Research Laboratory, Baylor College of Medicine

MERRILL M. MITLER, Ph.D.
Associate Director of Animal Sleep Research, Department of Psychiatry, Stanford University School of Medicine

ROBERT L. WILLIAMS, M.D.
D. C. Irene Ellwood Professor and Chairman of the Department of Psychiatry, Baylor College of Medicine

CONTENTS

INTRODUCTION

*Blest be the man who first invented sleep—a
cloak to cover all human imaginings, food to
satisfy hunger, water to quench thirst, fire to
warm cold air, cold to temper heat, and, lastly,
a coin to buy whatever we need.*

Cervantes: *Don Quixote* **II.**68

Freud opened up the area of the importance of dream
content, and for the past 60 years this has played an important part in psychiatric theory and practice. However,
only in the past decade has the average psychiatrist become
aware of the importance of the study of sleep *per se* and how
it may relate to psychiatric theory and practice. Most behavioral scientists have a vague concept that sleep will be
one of the more important areas of impending research and
learning and that "it is something about which we should
know more." This volume should serve as a valuable introduction and provide a foundation for more detailed study of
the topic. It might stimulate the reader to be alert to the
significant literature that will be forthcoming in the next
few years.

The American College of Psychiatrists devoted its symposium in Dallas, Texas, on April 29, 1972, to the study of
sleep. The symposium was developed by Doctor Shervert
Frazier, Program Chairman for the 1972 meeting. These

papers were presented at that symposium, the express purpose of which was to give the psychiatric clinician pragmatic information in the field of sleep research, emphasizing findings that might be useful in daily practice.

The field of sleep study represents a rapidly advancing frontier with applications not only for the treatment of everyday tensions but also for psychiatric illnesses and the entire field of medicine. Those who hope to find the definitive information they need for immediate clinical application will be disappointed, in part, as will those who expect to find ready made answers about the causes, effects, and significance of sleep. We hope that this book will be of aid to all clinicians. But it is not a book that one can read through once and expect to remember in detail, to integrate, understand, and promptly put to use in practice.

The first presentation, by William C. Dement, a pioneer and outstanding investigator in the field, and his colleague, Merrill Mitler, reviews the current neurophysiology and neurochemistry of sleep. This chapter is the most technical and difficult portion of the book, especially for the clinician unsophisticated regarding basic laboratory sciences as they relate to sleep studies. It provides basic and technical information, explaining the meaning and derivation of various terms and common uses, describing the phenomenology of sleep and wakefulness, and detailing underlying mechanisms believed to be responsible for, or associated with, phenomena involved in these areas.

Much of the basic research unavoidably has been performed on lower mammals, but Dement and Mitler discuss many findings which may be applicable to man, pointing out that some of the generalities apply across species. This presentation elaborates the fascinating historical developments in the field, even including the reasoning involved in a series of experiments, followed either by disappointment or reward at the outcome. An example of this is the discussion of a theoretical explanation of hallucinatory behavior, even though the original intricate experiments did not turn out as expected; after additional work some of this theory re-emerges as possibly compatible with the data.

Experimental evidence relating serotonin to non-REM sleep and catecholamines to REM sleep, the implications of the findings and the resulting theoretical construct of sleep mechanisms as they relate to clinical psychiatric disorders obviously all warrant further exploration. This paper concludes by raising the possibility that the data on anticholinergic effects may permit a reinterpretation of previous work with hallucinogens.

The chapter by Robert L. Williams and Ismet Karacan provides an orderly, thorough and complete listing of sleep disorders which describes an entire area, this time from a clinical human patient standpoint. They define and present relevant clinical data under four major headings: *Primary Sleep Disorders, Secondary Sleep Disorders, Parasomnias,* and *Sleep-Exacerbated Disorders.*

Williams and his colleagues, Wilse B. Webb and H. W. Agnew, did pioneer work that helped to establish the baseline electroencephalogram parameters of normal human sleep. Williams and Karacan have extended their early studies to include all ages of males and females, including females during each stage of the menstrual cycle as well as after the menopause and the post menopausal period. From these baseline studies, they have been able to establish that electroencephalograph sleep patterns are a function of age, sex, and the menstrual cycle.

Knowing what normal sleep is like has made it possible to examine the patterns in various sleep disorders and in clinical conditions of disordered sleep. Their findings and the findings of others constitute the essence of this presentation.

Their report and the chapter by Anthony and Joyce Kales that follows illustrate how sleep studies can be useful to the clinician in diagnosis and treatment.

Some of Williams and Karacan's topics were naturally of more interest to the psychiatrist than others; among these are the primary sleep disorders and those secondary to psychiatric conditions. Those especially interested in psychosomatic medicine will find many fascinating points in their section on sleep exacerbated disorders.

This paper is overwhelming if one considers merely the many possible combinations of the several sleep stages with the multiple symptom and disease combinations covered. Some idea of the breadth of coverage and the quality of scholarship represented in this article can be obtained from the very extensive list of 220 references.

The final chapter by Anthony and Joyce Kales also describes the diagnosis of sleep disturbances, with special emphasis on the management and treatment of these disorders. The authors note in detail their original studies of a variety of conditions, including somnambulism, enuresis, insomnia, asthma, peptic ulcer and hypothyroidism and, in each case, the diagnostic and treatment implications.

In addition, they discuss the etiology of insomnia, particularly the relationship of personality characteristics to insomnia, stressing the key role of depression which should be familiar to the clinician. They note the relationship of insomnia to personality characteristics as shown by Minnesota Multiphasic Personality Inventory profiles.

Reporting on their studies of many drugs, they make pragmatic recommendations to the practitioner in making the selection of therapeutic agents more rational. They attempt to bring order out of chaos concerning the utilization of drugs. Their concern regarding hypnotic drug dependence brings out important features of withdrawal symptoms,

nightmares and "accidental suicide." They emphasize re-
peatedly the strong influence of age in sleep patterns. They
also discuss psychotherapeutic approaches to insomnia carried out in conjunction with pharmacological treatment and
describe the problems and complexities arising in such a
combined therapeutic program.

Finally, the Kales devote a major portion of their presentation to discussing the consulting and educative efforts of
their Sleep Research and Treatment Facility. Their pragmatic recommendations for the diagnosis and therapy of
sleep disorders contain broad implications that have been
shown to be useful not only to the general physician but to
the Food and Drug Administration (FDA). Their work has
encouraged pharmaceutical firms and the FDA to include
sleep laboratory evaluations of hypnotic drugs as an important step in the total evaluation of the effectiveness of
these compounds. In addition, their work has favorably in-
fluenced the quality of advertising for these drugs.

These three presentations represent a progression from the
laboratory-animal-physiological level through encyclopedic-
enumerative-descriptive-clinical to the practical case level-
drug treatment-psychotherapy-general management levels.
Readers should be able to derive some immediate benefit in
management of individual cases. The authors have avoided
overstating their information and applications, and the
reader will not put down this book feeling that he has any-
where near the final understanding. Obviously, he will recog-
nize that sleep is an area which two to three decades ago
was mostly unknown and certainly had not received the
scientific investigation which it warranted. Knowledge was
anecdotal and speculative, and treatment was almost intui-
tive or impressionistic, to say the most.

The subject of sleep has seen an explosion of research and
knowledge. It is to be hoped that recent federal cutbacks

in funds for research will somehow be circumvented in this area, so that the capable research which has been started may be continued. With the current high level of interest, it seems certain that there will be important future developments and more aspects of this topic will become clear. We have some of the basic information and the clinician should continue to receive additional information, permitting him to take advantage of greater knowledge from sleep studies for diagnosis and treatment.

Studies of the relationship of physiological sleep to psychological states offer one of the finest opportunities for the understanding of the age old mind-body continuum. Perhaps no other area of human functioning is so squarely planted in this nether zone of fantasy thought perception and neurophysiological activity.

This book should further establish the fact of the importance of the study of sleep for modern medicine. The contributors have delineated precisely the state of our present knowledge, including the pitfalls of some concepts and areas where further research should be directed. The reader should be convinced, as Williams and Karacan point out, that if the treatment of many disorders is not based on the sleeping as well as the waking behavior of the patient, then it is only partial treatment.

One of the functions of the American College of Psychiatrists is to provide graduate education for its members as well as for psychiatrists in general. This volume brings an additional purpose of the College, which is to interest and involve non-psychiatric physicians as well as allied psychiatric disciplines in areas that not only are of interest to the psychiatrist but to the entire medical profession and to anyone interested in the more comfortable functioning of man.

GENE USDIN

SLEEP RESEARCH
AND
CLINICAL PRACTICE

1.

New Developments in the Basic Mechanisms of Sleep

WILLIAM C. DEMENT, M.D.
MERRILL M. MITLER, Ph.D.

MAMMALIAN EXISTENCE involves the temporal compartmentalization of behavior into three readily identifiable, behavioral states: wakefulness, NREM sleep and REM sleep. We are primarily interested in human sleep, but some of the generalities do apply across species.

There is good agreement among investigators that criteria of wakefulness are an activated EEG and signs of skeletal motor activity (best indicated by an active electromyogram). Non-rapid-eye-movement (NREM) sleep (also known as slow wave sleep) is defined by slow waves and spindles in the EEG; usually the subject is passively recumbent. Paradoxically, the tonic EMG activity of wakefulness

This research was supported by National Institute of Mental Health Grants MH 13860 and NS 10727, National Aeronautics and Space Administration Grant NGR 05-020-168, and Career Development Award MH 5804 to the first author. The second author was supported by National Institutes of Health Training Grant MH 8304. We also wish to acknowledge the invaluable contributions of Dr. Jack Barchas, who performed all biochemical analyses.

continues into slow wave sleep. Finally, we define REM sleep by noting an activated EEG, as in wakefulness; signs of nonreciprocal, generalized skeletal motor inhibition, specifically the absence of electromyographic activity in the neck muscles; and finally, superimposed on this, eye movements and other short-lasting events (phasic activity). We assume that phasic activities, including the cat PGO wave, are generated exclusively from within the brain. "REM," it should be noted, is a neurological term and has nothing to do with rapid eye movements. Animals without eyes have REM sleep.

The word "state" also needs further comment. State usually refers to a condition in which something exists that is qualitatively different from other possible conditions in which it may exist. A specific condition or state is usually recognized by the necessary presence of one or more attributes that are absent at all other times, or absent in a specific constellation. For example, when water exists in the frozen state it possesses attributes of solidity and rigidity that are present at no other time. In complex living organisms the taxonomic problem of defining states becomes to some extent a matter of consensus and judgment.

Also used in connection with sleep is the term "stage." "Stage" usually refers to a relatively precise but arbitrary subdivision in the course of the continuously progressing change in some variable. It is obvious from this that almost any number of stages may be defined within a state. However, with regard to NREM sleep, only four stages are commonly accepted as subdivisions. These are the EEG stages of NREM sleep. A confusing element has always existed in that the EEG during REM sleep has been called ascending Stage 1. This term is no longer used. The EEG during NREM Stage 1 and REM sleep are not exactly the same although misleadingly similar. There are no stage subdivisions of the REM state that have been widely accepted. To sum up, Stage 1 + Stage 2 + Stage 3 + Stage 4 equal NREM sleep. NREM sleep + REM sleep equals total sleep. It is difficult in non humans to define NREM stage subdivisions. However, Ursin (1968) has attempted to define two stages of NREM sleep in the cat on the basis of amount of slow waves. Our group informally designates two stages of NREM sleep on the basis of whether or not there are PGO spikes in subcortical recordings.

It may be useful at this point to penetrate deeper into the phenomenological aspects of the behavioral states. It is important to emphasize that the salient feature of wakefulness is the environmental engagement of the organism; he interacts with the world around him. The onset of slow wave sleep entails the cessation of such interaction. At the moment of sleep, the organism essentially stops perceiving much of his environment. Therefore, the significance of spindles and slow waves in the EEG may not be crucial, convenient though they are as "signs" of slow wave sleep. For example, suppose we ask an individual to sit with his eyes taped open and to make a motor response when a light flash is presented. At some point he will not respond to the flash. The moment of sleep is best defined as this point of perceptual disengagement. Immediately after such a failure the EEG patterns can still show wakefulness. Thus, we could conceivably abolish slow waves and spindles without abolishing the process of perceptual disengagement. Accordingly, we must acknowledge that it is not clear if slow waves and spindles are processes which really begin at the point of response inhibition and only build up enough to appear in the EEG a few minutes later, or are entirely separate and, perhaps, redundant processes. But until proven otherwise, we must continue to think of slow waves and spindles as meaningful, although often belated, signs of a central inhibitory state.

REM sleep, phenomenologically, may be considered as a behavioral anomaly. For mammals REM sleep may be sleep; it may be wakefulness; or it may be both. The forebrain appears to be aroused, there is EEG activation, elevated brain temperature, and so on. There appear to be two quite independent processes which accompany this arousal and thus prevent what we might ordinarily think of as wakefulness.

One of these is a process of tonic motor inhibition which has been well-studied by a number of workers (see Pompeiano, 1970, for an excellent review). The tonic inhibition is most conveniently measured by recordings of the electromyogram of the neck muscles. Most workers use the posterior neck muscles in the cat and the dygastric muscles in the human for such electromyography. EMG suppression is highly correlated with other measures of REM sleep and with other indicators of neural inhibition. The exact pattern of inhibition, while not totally understood, does seem to involve hyperpolarization of alpha motor neurons. There are many muscles which are not continuously inhibited during REM sleep. These include the diaphragm, the extra-ocular muscles, the middle ear muscles, the intercostal muscles, some muscles of the face, and of the nasal pharynx and larynx. Specific tests of inhibition have been done in the human and it is clear that reflex activity such as tendon reflexes are suppressed (Hodes and Dement, 1964). Pompeiano has studied these processes extensively in the cat and has proposed that there is tonic nonreciprocal inhibition of alpha motor neurons from pathways descending in the dorsal lateral funiculi. This REM associated nonreciprocal inhibitory process has been equated with the cataplectic attack of narcolepsy and it is possible that by observing this attack we can get a better notion of the overall pattern of inhibition. In cataplexy, voluntary movement, except the eyes, appears to be impossible when the attack is full-blown. However, there are many gradations and occasionally a cataplectic attack is experienced only as a momentary weakness or as an inability to move rapidly. In the full-blown attack, however, there is profound, frightening paralysis; such paralyses fortunately last only a few seconds. The nonreciprocal motor inhibition is of interest since it occurs spontaneously only during REM sleep and the pathological condition of cataplexy. In terms of a neuroanatomical substrate it has been known since the 1940's from the work of Magoun and Rhines (1946) that there is a system of neurons in the medial portion of the medullary reticular formation which if stimulated in a lightly anesthetized animal will produce nonreciprocal inhibition. A number of investigators have attempted to stimulate these areas in the waking animal and in this state nonreciprocal inhibition cannot be elicited. It is possible that this inhibitory center is the final common path of motor inhibition during REM sleep. Pathways impinging upon this area include a pathway originating in the orbital cortex, a pathway originating in, or passing through, the basal forebrain area, and a pathway from the nucleus locus coeruleus. The first two are implicated because stimulation of these areas in a lightly anesthesized animal will elicit nonreciprocal inhibition or sleep (Sauerland *et al.*, 1967; Sterman and Clemente, 1962a and 1962b). The locus coeruleus or subcoeruleus is implicated because Jouvet and Delorme (1965) have shown in a very dramatic series of experiments that bilateral lesions in this area will abolish motor inhibition during REM sleep. These experiments have since been confirmed by Henley and Morrison (1969). In terms of biochemistry, it is not clear whether or not any particular putative transmitter is specifically related to motor inhibition either in the final path or one of the paths impinging upon the medullary inhibitory area. Acetylcholine has often been implicated in motor inhibition (Cordeau *et*

al., 1963; George *et al.*, 1964; Hernandez-Peon *et al.*, 1967).
It is of some interest, however, that Vaughn *et al.* (1972)
found alpha-methylparatyrosine in humans increases REM
sleep while at the same time decreasing the motor inhibition.

The second process which accompanies the "arousal" of
REM sleep is called phasic activity during which the nervous
system emits bursts of activity. Such discharges may occur
through some phasic generator mechanism. Phasic activities
are short-lasting physiological events within REM sleep.
We feel that the central biphasic electrical phenomena, now
called the ponto-geniculo-occipital (PGO) wave, is the best
example. These waves are often equated with generator potentials, i.e., they are thought to be directly related to whatever center or system generates all phasic events from
muscle twitches to eye movements, including bursts of unit
discharge in various areas of the brain, cardiopulmonary
irregularities, phasic changes in pupil diameter, and so on.
However, we may legitimately ask whether or not the above
formulation is true. Perhaps PGO waves are just another
member of a larger class of phasic events. Indeed recent
work (Roffwarg, personal communication) with phasic middle ear muscle activity, first described by Baust *et al.* (1964)
and Dewson *et al.* (1965), suggests that phasic contractions
of middle ear muscles are not always coincident with PGO
spikes recorded from the lateral geniculate nucleus of the
cat, nor are they coincident with rapid eye movements in
the human. Also in humans, our observations on phasic inhibition of EMG activity (Pivik and Dement, 1970) and
Rechtschaffen's phasic integrated potential (Rechtschaffen
et al., 1972) indicate still another example of asynchrony in
phasic activity. Thus we may have one phasic generator
which elicits differential responses, or we may have several
phasic generators.

When both tonic inhibitory and phasic processes occur

simultaneously with arousal, we call it REM sleep. But an important point is that in the normal organism the simultaneity is far from absolute. At times, phasic activity or motor inhibition may accompany slow waves and spindles.

Returning to phenomenology now, let us assume for the sake of argument that the arousal processes characteristic of REM sleep (i.e., EEG activation, brain temperature elevation, etc.) are in fact identical to the arousal processes characteristic of behavioral wakefulness. Then, we may note that if we add only the process of nonreciprocal motor inhibition, we have what is called by physicians a state of cataplexy, wherein the patient cannot move, although he greatly desires to do so; and furthermore, wherein he is completely awake from the point of view of perceiving the external environment. If his eyes happen to be open, he sees; if there are sounds, he hears. If we add to wakefulness only the phasic process, we may postulate that we would have a waking dream or hallucinatory state.

There is some evidence supporting this line of reasoning. The fascinating, organized motor behavior in REM sleep of the locus coeruleus lesioned cat is one striking example of the similarity of REM sleep to wakefulness (Jouvet and Delorme, 1965; Henley and Morrison, 1969). One could say, then, that the occurrence of nonreciprocal inhibition plus phasic activity in wakefulness is the REM state.

Neural circuits definitely control wakefulness, NREM, and REM sleep, but the neurophysiological study of such circuits has not yielded the best explanation of control processes. The most active research area in recent years has been the neurochemistry of the monoamines and sleep. This is partly because more is known about these compounds and because better techniques of localization and estimating turnover are available. In terms of putative neural transmitters, acetylcholine has certainly enjoyed a great deal of attention, although this amine is not amenable to the techniques of histofluorescent localization.

The modern biochemistry of sleep may be said to have begun with Jouvet's observations on the reserpinized cat (see Jouvet, 1967). Jouvet found that depletion of monoamines leads to the disappearance of the states of sleep. He found that this effect was reversed by both 5-hydroxytryptophan, a precursor of serotonin, and by L-DOPA, the precursor of dopamine and noradrenalin. Jouvet suspected that serotonin had something to do with NREM sleep and catacholomines with REM sleep. At that time Swedish investigators were developing histofluorescence techniques which lead to the localization of serotonergic and catecholaminergic cells and their projections. It was then that Jouvet developed the serotonin hypothesis of NREM sleep on the basis of raphe lesion and neuropharmacological experiments; other studies had already implicated catecholamines, the pons, and nucleus locus coeruleus as crucial for REM sleep. Jouvet and his colleagues observed the effects of specific attacks upon serotonergic neurons (Jouvet, 1969). They achieved pharmacological specificity with acute administration of the serotonin depletor parachlorophenylalanine (PCPA) and anatomical specificity with stereotaxic lesions. Both of these attacks led to insomnia or a great reduction in total sleep time and the emergence of PGO activity in the waking state. Our studies focused on chronic PCPA administration. These data have been reported elsewhere (Dement *et al.*, 1972). Very briefly we found that PCPA reduced serotonin concentrations in all parts of the brain (zero to 10% of controls) by the fifth PCPA treatment day. During the first 24 hours after the beginning of PCPA administration, REM time generally stayed the same or increased. NREM was slightly reduced. Near the the end of the third day, total sleep time dropped precipitously and often reached zero for limited periods. Minima were generally seen on the fifth day of PCPA treatment. After two or three days of very low values a marked recovery in total sleep time began, reaching approximately 70% of the baseline values, even during continued administration of PCPA. At the point where total sleep time began to increase, reorganization in the temporal sequencing of the sleep states became apparent. In the intact cat, there is a marked tendency for the order of states to be wakefulness, then NREM, then REM sleep. In the chronic PCPA cat, the order was most typically wakefulness, then REM, then NREM sleep.

The earliest changes in phasic activity during PCPA administration were an increase in the rate of PGO spikes during REM sleep and a decrease in the number of spikes that commonly precede REM periods. These changes were evident within 8 to 12 hours after the first dose of PCPA.

We observed an emergence of PGO activity throughout NREM and the waking state. Such activity could be seen at each point in the pons-geniculate-occipital cortex circuit. As this activity appeared in the waking state, the overall rate of spike discharge began to drop in REM sleep. Accompanying PGO waves in the waking state were behavioral effects, such as orienting behavior which occurred during bursts of PGO waves.

During the period when PGO waves were discharging in the waking state, behavioral arousal or intense stimulation could block PGO activity. In addition, L-DOPA (10-15 mg/kg) or amphetamine (1 mg/kg) totally suppressed the PGO waves for variable lengths of time. 5-HTP totally reversed the release of PGO waves.

Thus, if we assume that the primary PCPA effect was inhibition of serotonin turnover, then the earliest and possibly the most basic effect of this change was on the regulation of

PGO spike discharge. Even after sleep returned PGO spike regulation did not return.

When we first began the study of chronic serotonin depletion in cats, we thought we had discovered an adequate alternative interpretation for the role of serotonergic neurons that would explain both the insomnia and the later return of sleep. This explanation was in terms of the major role being a regulation of phasic activity. The behavioral consequence of waking PGO waves was unquestionably arousing. A burst of PGO waves *always* evokes orienting if the animal is awake or even drowsy. Thus, we reasoned that PCPA leads to serotonin depletion which releases PGO waves which keep the animal awake just as would exogenous stimuli. We were impressed in our early studies by the close temporal association between the development of insomnia and the development of waking PGO waves. However, a closer analysis with larger numbers of cats showed that this was not entirely true. Clear cut insomnia could appear in the absence of waking PGO waves. However, we now know that phasic activity can occur in the absence of PGO waves. Thus it is possible that PGO waves are a delayed manifestation of disinhibition of phasic activity.

At any rate, the return of sleep on the eighth PCPA day may be understood as both a subsidence of the intensity of unregulated PGO waves and a simple habituation of the cat to this internal disturbance. Jouvet has postulated that the return of sleep represents a genuine recovery in serotonergic neurons, and suggests from the work of Pujol (Pujol et al., 1971) that tryptophan hydroxylase is only 80% inhibited at this time and that there is probably a micropool of serotonin which is functionally active. In the first place, the chronic PCPA animal is not normal: there is no regulation of PGO waves. Furthermore, sleep staging is reversed. Finally, a microscopic dose (0.5 mg/kg) of 5-HTP given at this time will immediately suppress waking PGO waves but will have no effect on sleep *per se*.

Since phasic activity and PGO waves are such prominent components of REM sleep, since REM sleep may be equated with the hallucinatory activity of dreaming, and since PGO waves and phasic activity seem to embody or represent an internal stimulation, it is reasonable that these events might be the neurophysiological substrate of hallucinatory behavior. Because of these considerations, we expected that the administration of hallucinogenic drugs and/or hallucinatory pharmacologic manipulation would be accompanied by a waking discharge of PGO waves as in the PCPA animal. This is not the case. We have administered LSD, dimethyl tryptamine, and, following the lead of Jones (1972), tropolone, a catechol-methyltransferase inhibitor plus L-DOPA, to cats. In every case hallucinatory behavior was produced, particularly in the latter, but in no case was this behavior accompanied by visible, eye-movement independent PGO waves.

We then turned our attention to possible mechanisms which regulate the occurrence of PGO activity. Since serotonin cells are concentrated in the brainstem raphe, Jacobs *et al.* (1972a) studied the effects of electrical stimulation of the raphe nuclei in the cat. Electrodes were implanted in raphe dorsalis, pontis, and magnus. When raphe dorsalis was stimulated during REM sleep, complete suppression of geniculate PGO waves occurred during the period of stimulation. Similar stimuli were ineffective in suppressing PGO waves when delivered to raphe pontis and raphe magnus. Stimulation of the dorsalis in the waking state produced little or no discernible behavioral effects, and when delivered to the sleeping animal, did not cause awakening. Thus the stimulation experiments are consistent with the notion that raphe dorsalis neurons might exert tonic inhibitory control over PGO waves and possibly other classes of phasic events except, of course, during REM sleep.

Jouvet and his colleagues have held that PGO waves depend upon catecholamines. One piece of evidence for this is that alpha-methyl-DOPA, which is metabolized to the false transmitter, alpha-methyl-noradrenaline and displaces noradrenaline from stores, suppresses PGO spike activity. There is also some evidence from electrolytic and chemical lesions in the locus coeruleus. The most damaging evidence against this notion are the several studies with alphamethyl-paratyrosine which selectively inhibits tyrosine hydroxylase and leads to a depletion of noradrenaline and dopamine (King and Jewett, 1971; Hartmann et al., 1971). This compound is nephrotoxic, however, and it is difficult to achieve total depletion, although turnover may indeed be stopped. In an effort to overcome this objection, Henriksen and Dement (1972) gave cats alphamethylparatyrosine by intravenous drip in a dosage calculated to be supramaximal and saw, as have other workers, a slight increase in NREM sleep or modest decrease in the amount of wakefulness, and an increase in the amount of REM sleep. Thus it is very difficult to attribute the PGO spike discharge to catecholaminergic neurons. To evaluate further the role of catecholamines in PGO activity, Jacobs et al. (1972 b) studied the PCPA treated cat in which waking PGO waves can be studied without contamination by other REM components. We regard waking PGO waves as homologous to those of REM sleep. Reasons for such an assumption are: a) As the number of waking PGO waves increases after PCPA treatment, the number of PGO waves decreases per REM sleep epoch. b) Following the discharge of a large number of PGO waves during a REM sleep period in a PCPA cat, waking waves only slowly reappear in the subsequent waking state. c) Both waking and REM sleep PGO waves frequently precede eye movements, while in the normal animal, lateral geniculate waves associated with eye movements always follow eye movements. d) Finally, both waking and REM sleep PGO waves are recorded unattenuated from leads in visual cortex when the animal is placed in the dark, while the size of cortical waves associated with waking eye movements diminishes.

After the PGO waves appeared in the waking state as the result of pretreatment with DL-PCPA, 150 mg/kg subcutaneously, the following presumptive norepinepherine receptor blockers were administered: Pimozide, 2.5 to 4.0 mg/kg; alpha-adrenergic blocker, phentolamine, 4.0 mg/kg; phenoxybenzamine, 7.5 to 10.0 mg/kg; beta-adrenergic blocker, propranalol hydrochloride, 4.0 mg/kg. The results were dramatically unequivocal. None of the four blocking agents had a significant effect on the rate of PGO wave discharge.

We then investigated the possible role of cholinergic mechanisms by giving the anticholinergic drug, atropine sulphate, to chronic PCPA cats. We found that this compound totally blocked the occurrence of PGO waves in doses as low as 0.25 mg/kg. This effect could be at least partially reversed by a subsequent injection of eserine. Evidence that the atropine effect was due to a direct effect on the central nervous system derives from the fact that equivalent doses of atropine methyl bromide, which does not cross the blood-brain barrier in significant quantities, had no effect on discharge rate of PGO waves. An observation worth noting is that the lowest dose of atropine which did suppress spikes did not produce the well-known EEG synchronization during the period of spike suppression.

Atropine's blocking of PGO activity was further substantiated in acute experiments. Unimplanted cats were pretested with 150 mg/kg DL-PCPA for 5 days. They were then anesthetized and placed in a stereotaxic apparatus which allowed deep electrodes to be positioned optimally for recording PGO activity from both pons and lateral geniculate. Once level of anesthesia was adjusted for optimal PGO discharge, drugs could be administered and evaluated. Effects on PGO waves of atropine, atropine methyl bromide, and eserine in these acute circumstances were similar to findings in chronic animals regardless of where PGO activity was recorded.

Atropine has been well-investigated in the intact animal (e.g. Wikler, 1952). It appears, however, that investigators have not dealt with REM sleep as a single process and have failed to rule out non-specific effects on REM sleep. This is a difficult problem in the intact animal. Henriksen et al. (1972 b) attempted to overcome this problem by prior potentiation of REM sleep to the point where its occurrence would override secondary effects. Any pharmacological manipulation utilized in the investigation of a behavioral state runs the risk of secondarily or non-specifically disrupting that state. For example, when atropine is administered to cats in high doses it results in medriasis, dryness of mouth, tachycardia and ataxia. Such effects may secondarily block the occurrence of REM sleep. Previous investigations have shown that when atropine has been administered to cats deprived of REM sleep, the ensuing predisposition for behavioral sleep overcomes the disruptive effects of the atropine treatment. Five animals were completely deprived of REM sleep for five days by means of a continuously moving treadmill, while minor amounts of NREM sleep could be obtained. At the end of the deprivation period the animals were placed in a recording chamber and allowed to go through two polygraphically monitored REM periods to act as controls. The animals were then given an injection of atropine sulphate (1.0 to 3.0 mg/kg) intraperitoneally, and the polygraphic recordings were continued for the next 6 to 12 hours. Atropine methyl-bromide in equivalent doses was also administered. The animals, in spite of atropine-excitement, would soon assume a recumbent position and enter NREM sleep. Later, 20 to 40 minutes after atropine administration, cervical muscle tone began to decrease concomitant with an increase in the frequency of discharge of PGO waves. This was soon followed by complete muscle atonia and a further increase in the discharge of PGO waves. Slow waves continued to appear in the cortical EEG although there was some attenuation in their amplitude and in the rate of occurrence of 12-14 Hz spindles. Bursts of rapid eye movements frequently occurred during these periods of atonia, but in contrast to control REM sleep periods, there was a marked decrease in the frequency of PGO waves associated with these eye movements. In fact, bursts of eye movements were frequently seen in the absence of any PGO waves, but such eye movements were associated with twitch-ing, fasciculation of the distal musculature and attenuation of EEG slow waves. On the other hand, isolated single eye movements were still associated with single PGO waves, typical of normal REM sleep episodes.

The electrophysiological effects following atropine sulfate were similar for all doses tested; however, higher doses (3 mg/kg) generally had a longer lasting period of action (up to 12 hours) as compared to lower doses.

When atropine methyl bromide was substituted for atropine sulfate, characteristic REM periods were observed, that is, desynchronized cortical EEG, complete muscle atonia, and bursts of PGO waves associated with bursts of eye movements.

These results in the intact cat underscore the role of acetylcholine. The first point is that atropine did not block REM sleep *per se*. Periodic atonia, as measured by cervical muscle tone, was unaffected by atropine administration. Furthermore, the atropine sulfate only affected bursts of PGO waves. It did not affect bursts of eye movements and distal muscular fasciculation, which were characteristically seen during these atonic episodes. Isolated PGO waves still occurred during the periods of muscular atonia.

These data on anticholinergic effects may permit a reinterpretation of our work with hallucinogens. The PGO wave-hallucination hypothesis may not be completely destroyed. In Jones' tropolone preparation, spikes were not coincident with hallucinatory episodes, but did appear somewhat later (Jones, 1972). Jones' observation plus our negative results with hallucinogenic drugs suggest two alternative interpretations. First, it may be that the types of hallucinations associated with PCPA-induced waking PGO waves are neurophysiologically different from those produced by tropolone plus L-DOPA and by known hallucinogens. However, it is just possible that phasic activity was indeed released by all compounds which produced hallucinatory behavior, but some accompanying effect blocked the appearance of PGO waves either temporarily as with tropolone or throughout the duration of drug effectiveness as with LSD.

REFERENCES

Baust, W., Berlucchi, G. and Moruzzi, G.: *Der einfluss von schlafund wachzustand auf den peripheren teil des auditorischen systemes. Pflueger Arch. Ges. Physiol.*, 281:15-16, 1964.

Cordeau, J., Moreau, A., Beaulines, A. and Laurin, C.: EEG and behavioral changes following microinjections of acetylcholine and adrenaline in the brainstem of cats. *Arch. Ital. Biol.*, 101:30-47, 1963.

Dement, W., Mitler, M. and Henriksen, S.: Sleep changes during chronic administration of parachlorophenylalanine. *Rev. Can. Biol.*, 31 (suppl): 239-246, 1972.

Dewson, J., Dement, W. and Simmons, F.: Middle ear muscle activity in cats during sleep. *Exp. Neurol.*, 12:1-8, 1965.

George, R., Haslett, W. and Jenden, D.: A cholinergic mechanism in the brainstem reticular formation: induction of paradoxical sleep. *Int. J. Neuropharmacol.,* 3:541-552, 1964.

Hartmann, E., Bridwell, T. and Schildkraut, J.: Alpha-methylparatyrosine and sleep in the rat. *Psychopharmacologia,* 21:157-164, 1971.

Henley, K. and Morrison, A.: Release of organized behavior during desynchronized sleep in cats with pontine lesions. *Psychophysiology,* 6:245, 1969.

Henriksen, S. and Dement, W.: Effects of chronic intravenous administration of 1-α methyl paratyrosine on sleep in the cat: a preliminary investigation. *Sleep Research,* 1:55, 1972.

Henriksen, S., Jacobs, B. and Dement, W.: Dependence of REM sleep PGO waves of cholinergic mechanisms. *Brain Res.,* 48:412-416, 1972.

Hernandez-Peon, R., O'Flaherty, J. and Mazzuchelli-O'Flaherty, A.: Sleep and other behavioral effects induced by acetylcholinic stimulation of basal temporal lobe and striate structures. *Brain Res.,* 4:243-267, 1967.

Hodes, R. and Dement, W.: Depression of electrically induced reflexes ("H-reflexes") in man during low voltage EEG "sleep." *Electroenceph. Clin. Neurophysiol.,* 17:617-629, 1964.

Jacobs, B., Asher, R., Henriksen, S. and Dement, W.: Electroencephalographic and behavioral effects of the electrical stimulation of the raphe nuclei in cats. *Sleep Research,* 1:23, 1972a.

Jacobs, B., Henriksen, S. and Dement, W.: Neurochemical bases of the PGO wave. *Brain Res.,* 48:406-411, 1972b.

Jones, B.: The respective involvement of noradrenaline and its deaminated metabolites in waking and paradoxical sleep. *Brain Res.,* 41:199-204, 1972.

Jouvet, M.: Neurophysiology of the states of sleep. *Physiol. Rev.,* 47:117-177, 1967.

Jouvet, M.: Biogenic amines and the states of sleep. *Science,* 163:32-41, 1969.

Jouvet, M. and Delorme, J.: *Locus coeruleus et sommeil paradoxal. C. R. Soc. Biol.,* 159:895-899, 1965.

King, C. and Jewett, R.: The effects of alpha-methyltyrosine on sleep and brain norepinepherine in cats. *J. Pharmacol. Exp. Ther.,* 177:188-195, 1971.

Magoun, H. and Rhines, R.: An inhibitory mechanism in the bulbar reticular formation. *J. Neurophysiol.,* 9:165-171, 1946.

Pivik, T. and Dement, W.: Phasic changes in muscular and reflex activity during non-REM sleep. *Exp. Neurol.,* 27:115-124, 1970.

Pompeiano, O.: Mechanisms of sensorimotor integration during sleep. *Prog. Physiol. Psychol.,* 3:1-179, 1970.

Pujol, J., Buguet, A., Froment, J., Jones, B. and Jouvet, M.: The central metabolism of serotonin in the cat during insomnia. A neurophysiological and biochemical study after administration of p-chlorophenylalanine or destruction of the raphe system. *Brain Res.*, 26:333-347, 1971.

Rechtschaffen, A., Michel, F. and Metz, J.: Relationship between extraocular and PGO activity in the cat. *Psychophysiol.*, 9:128, 1972.

Sauerland, E., Knauss, T., Nakamura, Y. and Clemente, C.: Inhibition of monosynaptic and polysynaptic reflexes and muscle tone by electrical stimulation of the cerebral cortex. *Exp. Neurol.*, 17:159-171, 1967.

Sterman, M. and Clemente, C.: Forebrain inhibitory mechanisms: cortical synchronization induced by basal forebrain stimulation. *Exp. Neurol.*, 6:91-102, 1962a.

Sterman, M. and Clemente, C.: Forebrain inhibitory mechanisms: sleep patterns induced by basal forebrain stimulated in the behaving cat. *Exp. Neurol.*, 6:103-117, 1962b.

Ursin, R.: The two stages of slow-wave sleep in the cat and their relation to REM sleep. *Brain Res.*, 11:347-356, 1968.

Vaughn, T., Wyatt, R. and Green, R.: Changes in REM sleep of chronically anxious depressed patients given alphamethylparatyrosine (AMPT). *Psychophysiol.*, 9:96, 1972.

Wikler, A.: Pharmacologic dissociation of behavior and EEG sleep patterns in dogs: morphine, N-allylmorphine and atropine. *Proc. Soc. Exp. Biol.*, 79:261-265, 1952.

2.

Clinical Disorders of Sleep

ROBERT L. WILLIAMS, M.D.
ISMET KARACAN, M.D., (Med.) D.Sc.

THOUSANDS OF MILES of sleep EEG data have been accumulated, and countless hours of effort have been expended by sleep researchers in many laboratories around the world. The degree of usefulness to the physician of the knowledge acquired depends upon its applicability to the solution of problems encountered in the day-to-day practice of medicine.

Considerable information has emerged from the sleep laboratories which can be useful to the physician. We will list and describe this information. For convenience, the clinically relevant data will be organized and presented under four major headings: Primary Sleep Disorders, Secondary Sleep Disorders, Parasomnias, and Sleep-Exacerbated Disorders.

This paper was developed while Drs. Williams and Karacan were members of the Department of Psychiatry, College of Medicine, University of Florida (Gainesville).

PRIMARY SLEEP DISORDERS

Primary sleep disorders are those in which disordered sleep is the only symptom and the only sign of abnormality. In this category we have included narcolepsy, cataplexy, chronic hypersomnia, the Kleine-Levin syndrome, the Pickwickian syndrome, isolated sleep paralysis, dream anxiety attacks, night terrors, and insomnia.

The term *narcolepsy* was first used by Gélineau in 1880 (73) to describe a condition of recurring, uncontrollable episodes of brief sleep. The symptom had been well-described in earlier reports (214) and had been recognized as early as Greco-Roman times (98).

Sleep attacks are often accompanied by auxiliary symptoms. Chief among these is cataplexy, which, according to Yoss and Daly (216), occurs in 68 percent of the cases. Cataplexy, which was first described by Loewenfeld (127) in 1902, is characterized by brief episodes of muscular weakness which are precipitated by laughter, anger, or other emotional excitement. The degree of disability may range in scope from a mere subjective feeling of weakness to almost total paralysis.

The "narcoleptic tetrad" (216) also includes the symptoms of sleep paralysis (an inability to move which occurs during the transitional period between sleep and wakefulness), and hypnagogic hallucinations (visual and auditory sensations which occur at sleep onset). Diplopia (31, 114), altered color vision (131), altered glucose tolerance (195), and decreased alcohol tolerance (79) have also been reported as symptomatic of narcolepsy.

The incidence of narcolepsy has been estimated at from 0.2 to 0.3 percent of the population (169). However, the syndrome may be more prevalent than was once suspected, since many cases probably continue to be misdiagnosed as hypothyroidism, hypoglycemia, or epilepsy (216). Yoss and Daly (216) have reported that 241 cases were seen at the Mayo Clinic between the years 1950 and 1954. In the absence of identifying auxiliary symptoms, an EEG examination, blood sugar and hormonal tests, x-rays and a neuropsychiatric evaluation are indicated as diagnostic aids prior to the prescription of antinarcoleptic agents.

Many recent EEG studies tend to discredit earlier notions of a relationship between narcolepsy and epilepsy (18, 40, 51, 71, 92). However, others continue to suggest a relationship to, or at least coincidence of, epilepsy in many patients (17, 35, 129, 174, 194, 207). Dynes and Finley (51) noted normal waking EEG's in subjects who had one or more auxiliary symptoms in addition to sleep attacks, but they found abnormal neurological signs and symptoms in patients who did not display auxiliary symptoms such as cataplexy. Daly and Yoss (40) emphasize that drowsiness and head-nodding in narcoleptics make interpretation of EEG records extremely difficult. In a study of 100 narcoleptics they reported finding only two grossly abnormal records when a proper basal point had been reached.

The possible etiological role of genetic, metabolic, and psychological factors is equally unclear. Krabbe and Magnussen (119) cited a total of 54 cases of familial narcolepsy reported in the literature prior to 1942. More recently Daly and Yoss (39) reported data from a large family in which narcolepsy was common. Most authors now reject a generalized metabolic etiology of narcolepsy (154, 159, 169, 217). Yoss and Daly (216) have stated that "no evidence exists that narcolepsy is of psychic origin." However, in a recent study of 22 patients, Mitchell et al. (141) found strong evidence of psychological stress and emotional imbalance as a precipitator of narcoleptic attacks. Other evidence (156, 195) lends support to this view.

Most sleep EEG research on the narcolepsy syndrome has attempted to relate that disorder to the REM state. REM sleep, besides being the period during which most dreaming occurs, is a period characterized by intense autonomic activity, including the inhibition of muscle tone (97) and spinal reflexes (95). The possible relationship to such narcoleptic symptoms as hypnogenic hallucinations and cataplexy is obvious. In examining the REM state in narcoleptics, researchers have uncovered some surprising results. In normals, the various stages of sleep occur in a regularly recurring, cyclical fashion. In almost every case, non-REM (NREM) sleep occurs first, with REM appearing after about 60-90 minutes of NREM sleep. Thereafter, REM and NREM alternate cyclically throughout the night. In many narcoleptics, REM occurs at, or soon after, the onset of sleep (93, 162, 172, 196, 209). Often the signs of sleep-onset REM are fewer than those of the complete REM constellation. For example, they may include loss of spinal reflexes (94) or the appearance of saw-tooth waves on the EEG (170), without the appearance of rapid eye movements or other REM phenomena.

It is interesting that REM disturbances are seen primarily in those narcoleptics who have auxiliary symptoms such as cataplexy or sleep paralysis. Patients suffering only sleep attacks rarely if ever exhibit sleep-onset REM periods (45, 172). Thus, the sleep EEG offers a neurophysiological test for distinguishing between narcoleptic patients who manifest only sleep attacks and those manifesting both sleep attacks and cataplexy, sleep paralysis, or hypnagogic hallucinations. As pointed out earlier, Dynes and Finley (51) were also able to differentiate between these two broad symptom types on the basis of clinical waking EEG's. Sixteen of seventeen patients who had both sleep attacks and cataplexy had normal EEG's. Patients with abnormal EEG's or other neurological signs for the most part suffered only sleep attacks. Therefore, while modern electroencephalography has not yet provided clearcut answers about the mechanisms or etiology of narcolepsy, it has provided some interesting information about the phenomena which precede and accompany narcolepsy attacks. The biochemistry and pharmacological treatment of narcolepsy are still largely unexplored areas.

Hypersomnia is characterized by a tendency to sleep for excessively long periods, either as an extension of nocturnal sleep into the late morning or past noon, or at various times during normal hours of wakefulness.

Unlike narcoleptics, patients with hypersomnia do not display the auxiliary symptoms of cataplexy, sleep paralysis or hypnagogic hallucinations. The tendency to sleep is not as irresistible, and hypersomniacs rarely complain of disturbed nocturnal sleep.

Hypersomnia may be either chronic or periodic. Periodic hypersomnia, which includes the Kleine-Levin and Pickwickian syndromes, will be discussed following a brief consideration of chronic hypersomnia. (This classification system is used for convenience. No attempt will be made in this paper to justify it on the basis of intrinsic coherence.)

A chronic tendency to sleep excessively may be associated with various disorders of the central nervous system, such as skull trauma, brain tumors or cerebrovascular disorders (147, 171), or it may occur in the absence of other recognizable pathology. Rechtschaffen and Roth (161) conducted a polygraph study of so-called "functional" hypersomnia, and reported some surprising results. They found that the sleep of hypersomniacs did not differ from that of normals in either cyclic regularity of stages or in percentages of sleep stages. They also found that heart and respiratory rates of hypersomniacs were significantly higher than those of normals, good sleepers, poor sleepers, and light sleepers. This was true both before, during, and after sleep. Rechtschaffen and Dement (159) have noted that hypersomniacs exhibit "postdormital confusion." These data indicate that excessive sleep, even in "functional" hypersomniacs in whom no other gross pathology can be seen, may be a mere manifestation of an underlying psychophysiological disturbance. The mechanism and etiology of the disturbance have yet to be demonstrated. It may be that a central psychophysiological disturbance is common to other chronic or periodic manifestations of hypersomnia.

Kleine (116) and Levin (125a, 125b) first described a clinical pattern characterized by "periodic somnolence and morbid hunger." Critchley and Hoffman (38) later named this disorder the *Kleine-Levin syndrome,* and Critchley (37) reported the chief characteristics to be "periodic hypersomnia and megaphagia in adolescent males." According to Critchley (37), in "genuine" cases the attacks first appear during adolescence, occur periodically at about six-month intervals, and eventually disappear spontaneously. Cases matching Critchley's original description are apparently quite rare (37, 190). A number of cases have been described in recent years (20, 52, 54, 69, 76, 200); however, a careful study reveals that many of these cases do not strictly conform to Critchley's original criteria. Duffy and Davison (50) recently reported finding a female case.

Few polygraph reports are available on daytime or nocturnal sleep characteristics of Kleine-Levin patients. Critchley (37) and Bonkalo (20) claim that the sleep of these patients during a daytime attack is normal. Thacore *et al.* (200) discuss these claims and point out that the presence of alpha activity and the absence of spindles would tend to contradict this conclusion. A number of other investigators have reported finding marked abnormalities in sleep EEG's during the daytime attacks (14, 54, 80, 200), as well as in the nocturnal sleep (14) of Kleine-Levin patients. Green and Cracco (80) report daytime sleep during attacks to be characterized by a slowing of background activity and generalized high-voltage, slow activity alternating with low-voltage, fast activity, with an absence of spindles. Barontini and Zappoli (14) have described nocturnal sleep as being considerably unstable in the various sleep stages.

Burwell *et al.* (27) first applied the label *Pickwickian syndrome* to a condition characterized by obesity, an enormous appetite, impaired respiration, fainting, and an often irresistible tendency to fall asleep. The condition had been described in the earlier literature under various names (12, 115, 182, 192). Drachman and Gumnit (49) were the first to study simultaneously the sleep pattern and respiratory characteristics of Pickwickian patients, and their results have been confirmed and elaborated by other workers (26, 33, 72, 74, 99, 120, 130, 157, 180, 199). From these studies it is now known that apneic intervals lasting from five to 60 seconds begin to appear very soon after the Pickwickian patient goes to sleep. Toward the end of each interval, EEG signs of arousal, such as K-complexes or alpha activity, appear and are soon followed by the return of respiration in the form of several deep breaths. The EEG arousal response is usually followed by light sleep patterns rather than a frank awakening, although the latter occurs periodically throughout the night. During successive apneic intervals, sleep patterns become progressively deeper, and the apneic intervals lengthen as sleep deepens.

As a result of this pattern of EEG and respiratory changes, the primary characteristic of the Pickwickian patient's sleep is its discontinuity. Thus, it is the summation of many short sleep periods which results in the Pickwickian patient's obtaining over ten hours of sleep per 24 hours (33, 72).

Furthermore, many patients exhibit little or no slow-wave or REM sleep (33, 72, 99, 147, 157, 199), and if REM periods do occur, they may be abnormally short (33, 99).

Some evidence (49, 60, 157, 177) suggests disturbed pulmonary function in Pickwickian patients, but in other patients pulmonary function is essentially normal (72). Obesity appears not to play a primary pathogenic role in the syndrome (120, 130). It has been noted (99) that the respiratory disturbances of the Pickwickian patient are exaggerations of disturbances which occur during normal sleep. Most authors (33, 99, 130), though not all (72), maintain that the Pickwickian patient's apnea is of central origin.

Chronic CO_2 hyposensitivity is postulated by some investigators (49, 99) to dispose the patients to diurnal sleep attacks in the absence of arousing stimuli. Others (72) have suggested that diurnal sleepiness is either the result of poor nocturnal sleep or a reflection of a primary disturbance in sleep-waking mechanisms.

Sleep paralysis as an isolated disorder has been found to occur in from 2% (78) to 15% (57) of groups surveyed. It appears to predominate in males, and there is occasionally a family history. Various psychiatric (122, 178, 204) and organic (2, 22, 23, 40, 41, 55, 56, 78, 216) explanations have been advanced to account for this phenomenon. EEG studies of isolated sleep paralysis attacks are virtually non-existent, but sleep paralysis episodes in narcoleptics seem to occur during sleep-onset REM periods (93, 171). Narcoleptics (94), like normal subjects (95), lost spinal reflexes during REM sleep, and the early portions of their sleep-onset REM periods appear to consist of lighter sleep than the drowsy state, later parts of the sleep-onset REM period, and later REM periods (93). It has been suggested (171) that sleep paralysis in its isolated form and in narcoleptics involves the occurrence of the muscular inhibition characteristic of REM sleep against a background of relative awareness.

EEG studies (24, 65) suggest that there are two types of frightening dreams—*night terrors* (pavor nocturnus and incubus attacks) and *dream anxiety attacks*. Both occur in all ages and cultures (132), but dream anxiety attacks are much more frequent (65). The latter are generally much milder than night terrors, and occur following a well-developed dream sequence during REM sleep. Awakenings from dream anxiety attacks are frequently, but not always, preceded by autonomic anxiety symptoms (65). Awakenings from night terrors occur predominantly from slow-wave sleep, are extreme panic reactions, and are accompanied and followed by large autonomic reactions (24, 65). Mental confusion is a prominent sign immediately after awakening, and this has led Broughton (24) to classify night terrors with sleepwalking and enuresis as a slow-wave sleep arousal phenomenon in individuals physiologically predisposed to display the disorder. Fisher *et al.* (65) suggest that REM dreams are mechanisms for modulating anxiety and desomatizing the physiological response to it, while the stage 4 night terror represents a failure of the ego to control anxiety.

Insomnia—inability to fall asleep, frequent and prolonged awakenings, early morning awakenings, in the absence of gross physical or psychological pathology—is probably one of the most common sleep disturbances. It has often been considered a symptom of some more basic pathology (109), but recent sleep EEG studies indicate that there is a physiological basis for the insomniac's complaint. We have found (111) these patients to have significantly longer sleep latencies, shorter sleep times, and less efficient sleep. Surprisingly, they averaged no more awakenings than age-matched controls. There was a suggestion that insomniacs establish a higher level of REM sleep than controls. We have also found

(107) that insomniacs are a significantly more heterogeneous group than controls on some sleep variables, suggesting several sub-types of primary insomnia, and that they vary more from one night to the next than controls. In addition, in some patients we have observed a superimposition of alpha activity on slow-wave sleep delta activity. These results have led us to speculate that extended sleep latency is sufficient to produce the insomniac's impression of having slept very little. On the other hand, excess REM sleep activation or abnormally distributed alpha activity may provide faulty feedback to patients who insist they do not sleep at all, regardless of objective evidence to the contrary. It may also be that the unpredictability of the insomniac's sleep from night to night contributes to his dissatisfaction with his sleep.

SECONDARY SLEEP DISORDERS

Secondary sleep disorders are those in which chronic clinical problems are accompanied by specific or non-specific sleep disturbances. In this category we have placed depression, schizophrenia, alcoholism, anorexia nervosa, hypothyroidism, and renal insufficiency.

The first EEG sleep study of a group of *depressed patients* predates the discovery of REM sleep. In 1946, Diaz-Guerrero *et al.* (46) described six manic-depressive patients in the depressed phase. These patients exhibited prolonged sleep latency, more frequent awakenings, an increased number of shifts between stages and "a greater proportion of sleep which is light." Since that time, depressed patients have been studied by many investigators (81, 82, 88-90, 136-140, 149, 186-189, 220).

Certain patterns in the sleep disturbances accompanying depression have been discovered. Most investigators agree that depressed patients have less total sleep time, less slow-wave sleep, and more awakenings during the night than normal subjects (82, 90, 91, 136-140, 149, 189, 220).

The picture with regard to the nature of REM sleep in depression is less clear. Many investigators have observed decreased REM sleep during the most severe stages of the illness, followed by an increase in this stage during the period of clinical improvement (82, 90, 91, 188, 189). However, Green and Stajduhar (81) reported a nearly normal percentage of REM time during the psychotic phase and Oswald et al. (149) reported no significant difference in REM time between patients and controls. The report of Oswald and co-workers (149) is difficult to assess because of the possible residual effects of medication administered during the course of the study.

There is also some evidence of abbreviated REM latencies (81, 89, 188), of shorter intervals between REM periods (188), and of an intensification of the phasic components of REM during the most severe stages of depression (188). Snyder (188), in noting this evidence, has suggested that a REM debt may be part of the causal developments leading to the psychotic phase of the depression and preceding clinical improvement. As will be discussed below, researchers have also been attracted to a REM debt theory of schizophrenia.

The discovery of REM sleep (11) and of its relationship to dreaming (44) provided the first major breakthrough for the empirical research of earlier theoretical notions concerning *schizophrenia*. Dement's (43) subsequent demonstration of a compensatory "need" for REM sleep after experimental deprivation seemed to further emphasize the possible importance of this stage in relation to the development of schizophrenic hallucinations.

The first EEG-EOG studies of REM sleep in schizophrenia

disclosed that there was no significant difference between REM time in schizophrenics and normal controls (42, 118). Despite the lack of empirical evidence, some investigators were tempted to hypothesize that schizophrenic symptoms might represent an intrusion of the REM state into wakefulness (64). It has been generally agreed (188, 208, 218) that if schizophrenia does indeed represent an intrusion of REM into wakefulness, there should be some evidence of REM "pressure" or REM deprivation in schizophrenic patients. Therefore, validation of the REM intrusion hypothesis is dependent upon a demonstration of decreased REM time, abbreviated REM latencies or increased frequency of the phasic components of REM during the acute psychotic stage, and perhaps compensatory rebound of REM time and a normalization of other REM parameters during remission, since these characteristics are seen in experimental REM deprivation (43, 102).

Some investigators have reported significantly reduced REM time in acute schizophrenics in the early part of their illness (121, 189). However, others continue to report no significant differences in REM time between schizophrenics and normal controls (28, 146, 193, 206, 210). Stern and associates (193) and Vincent and associates (206) have reported significantly abbreviated REM latencies during the acute psychotic phase; however, Kupfer *et al.* (121) reported significantly prolonged REM latencies during this period. Feinberg *et al.* (62) noted that, while the mean latency to REM of their schizophrenic patients was not significantly different from that of normal controls, REM latency values were either extremely abbreviated or extremely prolonged, i.e., bimodal, in the schizophrenics. Eye movement activity has been reported to be both noticeably higher in one study (85) and significantly lower in another study (63) of schizophrenics, when compared to normal controls.

Feinberg and associates (62) did note, however, that eye movement activity was significantly greater in hallucinating schizophrenics, as compared to non-hallucinating patients.

Differences in recording and scoring procedures could account for some of the inconsistencies in reported REM characteristics of schizophrenics. However, the statistically significant, but opposite, results reported by so many investigators would seem to be indicative of differences in degree and/or type and/or duration of the illness process.

Recent studies have shown that there is one sleep EEG characteristic which seems to be common to most schizophrenics. Caldwell and Domino (28) reported significantly reduced slow-wave sleep in schizophrenics. This finding has been confirmed by others (61, 121). This abnormality is apparently not specific to schizophrenia, but may be characteristic of most somato- and psychopathological disorders in which disturbed sleep is a prominent symptom. It was recently demonstrated (128) that schizophrenics also have difficulty in incrementing slow-wave sleep after prolonged (85 hours) total sleep deprivation. Interestingly, this inability to compensate slow-wave sleep has not been reported in other psychopathological groups in which reduced slow-wave sleep is a common characteristic. This suggests the possible presence in schizophrenics of an irreversible defect in brain synchronizing mechanisms.

Serious sleep disturbances are associated with prodromal and acute stages of the *alcoholic psychoses*. Slow-wave sleep and REM sleep appear to be suppressed during acute alcoholization (83). Initially there is an increase in slow-wave activity and a decrease in REM. Later both may disappear completely. Complete suppression of REM may be the precipitator of the seizures characteristic of this disorder. Withdrawal of alcohol is accompanied by rebounds of both slow-wave and REM sleep. The REM rebound may provide the basis for the hallucinations characteristic of withdrawal, while slow-wave sleep rebound may be related to the duration of the acute disease state. Gross and Goodenough (83) suggest that a sudden and large slow-wave sleep rebound is linked clinically to the so-called terminal sleep, which is typically followed by a clearing of the psychosis. When the slow-wave sleep returns more slowly, the recovery phase may be longer.

Patients suffering from *anorexia nervosa* show severe weight loss due to carbohydrate starvation. Crisp *et al.* (36) found that such patients show decreased total sleep time and amounts of stages 3, 4, and REM, increased amounts of stages 0 and 1, and increased latencies to onset of stages 1 REM and 3 prior to treatment, when compared to post-treatment values. The authors concluded that in these patients changes in sleep are more closely related to changes in nutritional status than to changes in emotional state. EEG sleep patterns are also significantly changed in *hypothyroid patients* (101), for they show reductions in stages 3 and 4 sleep. When dessicated thyroid treatment is instituted, these stages increase toward normal levels. Patients suffering from *chronic renal insufficiency* and treated with renal hemodialysis have been noted to experience insomnia at night (77, 179), and sleep EEG studies have shown definite sleep disturbances prior to dialysis (110, 150). Dialysis has been found to improve various aspects of sleep patterns to a greater or lesser extent (110, 150).

PARASOMNIAS

Parasomnia phenomena are those in which activity similar to waking behavior appears during sleep. We have included sleepwalking, sleep talking, bruxism (teethgrinding), and enuresis (bedwetting) in this category.

Sleepwalking occurs primarily in males (191) and is

quite often accompanied by enuresis and/or night terrors. Sleep EEG work has shown that sleepwalking typically occurs during slow-wave sleep (24, 96). Forced awakening of sleepwalkers from slow-wave sleep is accompanied by mental confusion (24, 104). Induced somnambulism in sleepwalkers and normal children is accompanied by diffuse and rather high amplitude EEG alpha activity, or low-voltage delta and beta activity without spindles (24). In the psychiatric literature sleepwalking has been considered an immature habit pattern or simple dissociation (5, 123, 124, 126, 135, 145, 175, 191), and the acting out of a dream or fantasy or the re-enactment of an earlier trauma (191). Cerebral metabolic disorder (153) and epilepsy (3) are other suggested etiologies. Broughton (24) proposed that sleepwalking is a slow-wave sleep arousal phenomenon in individuals who are physiologically predisposed to be aroused into sleepwalking.

Sleep talking appears to be quite common (32, 106, 148), whether as an isolated phenomenon (117, 148, 185) or as an accompaniment to other sleep (191, 198, 203), psycho-pathological (6, 19, 29), or organic (84, 211) disorders. Most sleep EEG evidence indicates that sleep talking usually accompanies body movements and occurs predominantly during NREM sleep (8, 34, 70, 105, 148, 160), although there do appear to be individuals whose sleep talking occurs predominantly or exclusively during REM sleep (9, 197). Sleep-talking incidents seem to be evenly distributed throughout the night (160). Arkin and his associates (7, 9) have found high concordance between content of sleep talking and content elicited on awakening from REM sleep-talking episodes. These latter results are of obvious interest since sleep talking may represent a more "pure" source of information about mentation during REM sleep.

Nocturnal enuresis refers to bedwetting in individuals old enough to have acquired control of micturition. It is most often seen in children and young adults (24), predominates in males (1), and may be a familial disorder (13, 86). Bedwetting typically occurs during slow-wave sleep (24, 47, 155). Bedwetters exhibit excessive bladder contractions throughout sleep (25) and have higher heart rates than normals throughout sleep, even during slow-wave sleep (24). Etiological theories of enuresis are numerous and varied: genetic, maturational, pathological, psychological, and habit deficiency etiologies have been proposed (213). Broughton (24) has suggested that enuresis is also a slow-wave sleep arousal phenomenon, as are sleep walking and night terrors, and that it therefore has similar characteristics.

Bruxism, or nocturnal teethgrinding, is bothersome both in the noise it produces and because of its damage to teeth and supporting structures (142, 166). There is strong evidence that diurnal and nocturnal teethgrinding are separate phenomena (165). Up to 15% of the individuals surveyed have given histories of bruxism, and males seem to be slightly more affected (163-166). The latest sleep EEG evidence indicates that bruxism occurs primarily during stage 2 sleep, and that bruxists show no disturbances in the distribution or amount of the various sleep stages (166, 176). EEG signs of arousal typically accompany the teethgrinding, and sound stimuli during sleep can provoke teethgrinding (176). Genetic habit patterns (58, 59), dental factors (53, 158), lesions of the brain stem or cortex (133, 152) and psychological factors (67, 68, 87, 142, 181, 201, 205, 212) are suggested etiologies. Others have proposed that bruxism is a partial arousal phenomenon (165, 166, 176) and that it occurs if the dopaminergic nigrostriatal system excessively drives the brain areas controlling jaw movement during the transition from sleep to wakefulness (176).

SLEEP-EXACERBATED DISORDERS

Sleep-exacerbated disorders are chronic clinical syndromes which are aggravated during sleep. A rather long list of cardiovascular, respiratory, neuromuscular, metabolic, and miscellaneous disorders fits into this category, and we will briefly discuss several of them.

Nocturnal angina pain attacks appear to occur predominantly during REM sleep (144), and we have shown angina patients to be quite different from each other in their sleep patterns (112). *Myocardial infarctions* frequently occur during sleep, and our preliminary studies indicate that infarct patients, when maintained on an intensive-care ward, are sleep-deprived due to the necessary therapeutic procedures or to pain. Their PVCs seem to increase during or immediately following REM periods. Increased hemolysis during sleep is a characteristic of the fatal *paroxysmal nocturnal hemoglobinuria* (134). The increase in plasma volume and the shift of blood from the lower extremities to the pulmonary circulatory system on assumption of the supine position are causes of the left ventricular failure and pulmonary edema which characterize *paroxysmal nocturnal dyspnea* (184). Paroxysmal disorders of the cranial arteries at night are implicated in *paroxysmal nocturnal,* or *cluster, headaches* (184).

In *emphysema* patients, abnormal increases in alveolar CO_2 tension (168) and decreases in arterial oxygen saturation (202) during sleep may contribute to these patients' post-awakening difficulties. *Asthmatics* typically have attacks at night, and EEG studies have shown children and adult asthmatics to have shorter sleep times and decreased stage 4 sleep (100, 103). In children, attacks are confined to the last two-thirds of the night, while in adults they occur throughout the night (100, 103).

Among the neuromuscular symptoms, *restless legs syndrome,* consisting of parasesia and restless legs primarily at night (21), affects younger age groups and pregnant women (184). Middle aged women are predominant sufferers of *acroparasthesia* (carpal tunnel syndrome), which is nocturnal pain, tinglings and numbness of the digits (184), and of *tired arm syndrome* (66), characterized by nocturnal pain and weakness of the forearm and hand. Males are primary sufferers of *familial periodic paralysis* (184), which consists of episodes of muscular weakness and eventual flaccid paralysis. Attacks usually begin at night, presumably because of an exaggeration of the normal loss of plasma potassium to the muscles during sleep (4, 219), and the resulting decrease in muscle membrane excitability. The elderly are most susceptible to *nocturnal pseudo-hemiplegia,* a numbness and immobility of one arm or side of the body. It may be some form of pressure palsy (184). Increasing age also predisposes to *night cramps* (184). Pregnant women appear to be particularly susceptible to acroparasthesia, restless legs, and night cramps, and calcium deficiency is the suspected etiology of the latter in these women (184). *Nocturnal myoclonus,* or frequent and repetitive jerks of the body or limbs, often with hypnogogic hallucinations, is said to occur only during light sleep and may be an arousal response to external stimuli or a temporary re-excitation of the reticular activating system (184).

Extensive evaluation of the sleep EEG as a diagnostic tool in the study of *epilepsy* has established that the EEG is more likely to be abnormal during sleep than during the waking state in known epileptics, particularly the psychomotor epileptic (75, 151, 215). Further studies have attempted to specify the relationships between the various stages of sleep and the types of seizure discharges (30, 113, 151). Different types of discharge do appear to favor certain stages, but at present there are many contradictions in the results. Nevertheless, it is almost certain that the sleep EEG can and will contribute significantly to our understanding of the biochemistry, neurophysiology, and pharmacology of the epilepsies.

The metabolic disorders *diabetes mellitus* and *rheumatoid arthritis* are also exacerbated during sleep. In the former there are abnormally wide variations in blood sugar concentrations during sleep (167). A loss of early morning peaks of plasma corticosteroids may be correlated with the rheumatoid arthritic's morning stiffness (167).

In *duodenal ulcer* patients the high nocturnal secretion rate of gastric acid is particularly exaggerated during REM sleep (10). *Painful nocturnal penile erections* (108), *nocturnal proctalgia*, or pain seeming to arise from the rectum (48), and *parasitic periodicity* (167) are other disorders which flare up during sleep. And finally, despite the facts that over 300 anti-snoring devices are registered in the U.S. patent office, and that an estimated 21 million sufferers blithely inflict their grunts, wheezes, buzzes and snorts on another 21 million spouses, snoring has not yet been studied in the sleep laboratory. However, it has been ascribed to a variety of physical and psychological causes.

The preceding discussion should amply testify to the fact that the study of sleep has a place in modern medicine. We now have a fairly solid neurophysiological description of many sleep phenomena, but it is also evident that we know virtually nothing about the sleep physiology of others. Nevertheless, the data we now have are sufficient to demonstrate that sleep is a state of changing levels of consciousness, and when we consider the manner in which sleep affects, or is affected by, disease states, we must be very careful to specify which type of sleep we are discussing. This will be a crucial distinction in future research, for in many areas sleep researchers are ready to tackle the question of why a particular disorder has a specific effect on a particular stage of sleep. And attempts to answer this question will most certainly involve more and more sophisticated biochemical and pharmacological approaches to the problem. The results of such studies will have an even greater influence on the physician than have any of the results reported so far, because they will provide a truly rational basis for treatment of patients. And surely this discussion cannot fail to convince us that if the treatment of many disorders is not based on the sleeping as well as the waking behavior of the patient, then it is only partial treatment.

REFERENCES

1. Agarwal, H. C., Mohan, D., and Mukerji, D. P.: Eneuresis. An etiological and therapeutic review. *Indian J. Med. Sci.,* 21:668-675, 1967.
2. Aird, R. B., Gordon, N. S., and Gregg, H. C.: Use of phenacemide (phenurone) in treatment of narcolepsy and cataplexy. A preliminary report. *Arch. Neurol. Psychiatry,* 70:510-515, 1953.
3. Aird, R. B., Venturini, A. M., and Spielman, P. M.: Antecedents of temporal lobe epilepsy. *Arch. Neurol.,* 16:67-73, 1967.
4. Aitken, R. S., Allott, E. N., Castleden, L. I. M., and Walker, M.: Observations on a case of familial periodic paralysis. *Clin. Sci.,* 3:47-57, 1937.
5. Allen, I. M.: Somnambulism and dissociation of personality. *Br. J. Med. Psychol.,* 11:319-331, 1932.
6. Andriani, G.: Fisiologia psicologia del sonniloquio. *Ann. Neurol.* (Torino), 10:299-308, 1892.
7. Arkin, A. M.: Sleep-talking: A review. *J. Nerv. Ment. Dis.,* 143: 101-122, 1966.
8. Arkin, A. M., and Reiser, M. F.: Experimentally produced sleeptalking as a method of sampling sleep ideation. Paper presented at the Annual Meeting of the Association for the Psychophysiological Study of Sleep, Palo Alto, California, 1964.
9. Arkin, A. M., Toth, M. F., Baker, J., and Hastey, J. M.: The frequency of sleep talking in the laboratory among chronic sleep talkers and good dream recallers. *J. Nerv. Ment. Dis.,* 151:369-374, 1970.

10. Armstrong, R. H., Burnap, D., Jacobson, A., Kales, A., Ward, S., and Golden, J.: Dreams and gastric secretions in duodenal ulcer patients. *New Physician*, 14:241-243, 1965.

11. Aserinsky, E., and Kleitman, N.: Regularly occurring periods of eye motility, and concomitant phenomena, during sleep. *Science*, 118: 273-274, 1953.

12. Auchincloss, J. H., Cook, E., and Renzetti, A. D.: Clinical and physiological aspects of a case of obesity, polycythemia and alveolar hypoventilation. *J. Clin. Invest.*, 34:1537-1545, 1955.

13. Bakwin, H.: Enuresis in children. *J. Pediatr.*, 58:806-819, 1961.

14. Barontini, F., and Zappoli, R.: A case of Kleine-Levin syndrome. Clinical and polygraphic study. In Gastaut, H., Lugaresi, E., Berti Ceroni, G., and Coccagna, G. (Eds.), *The Abnormalities of Sleep in Man*. Bologna: Aulo Gaggi, 1968, pp. 239-245.

15. Birchfield, R. I., Sieker, H. O., and Heyman, A.: Alterations in blood gases during natural sleep and narcolepsy. A correlation with the electroencephalographic stages of sleep. *Neurology* (Minneap.), 8: 107-112, 1958.

16. Birchfield, R. I., Sieker, H. O., and Heyman, A.: Alterations in respiratory function during natural sleep. *J. Lab. Clin. Med.*, 54:216-222, 1959.

17. Bjerk, E. M., and Hornisher, J. J.: Narcolepsy: A case report and a rebuttal. *Electroencephalogr. Clin. Neurophysiol.*, 10:550-552, 1958.

18. Blake, H., Gerard, R. W., and Kleitman, N.: Factors influencing brain potentials during sleep. *J. Neurophysiol.*, 2:48-60, 1939.

19. Bleuler, E.: *Lehrbuch der Psychiatrie*, 4th ed. Berlin: Springer, 1923, p. 88.

20. Bonkalo, A.: Hypersomnia. A discussion of psychiatric implications based on three cases. *Br. J. Psychiatry*, 114:69-75, 1968.

21. Bornstein, B.: Restless legs. *Psychiatr. Neurol.* (Basel), 141:165-201, 1961.

22. Brain, W. R.: Sleep: Normal and pathological. *Br. Med. J.*, 2:51-53, 1939.

23. Brock, S., and Wiesel, B.: The narcoleptic-cataplectic syndrome—an excessive and dissociated reaction of the sleep mechanism—and its accompanying mental states. *J. Nerv. Ment. Dis.*, 94:700-712, 1941.

24. Broughton, R. J.: Sleep disorders: Disorders of arousal? *Science*, 159:1070-1078, 1968.

25. Broughton, R. J., and Gastaut, H.: Further polygraphic sleep studies of enuresis nocturna (intra-vesical pressure). *Electroencephalogr. Clin. Neurophysiol.*, 16:626, 1964.

26. Bruhova, S., Nevsimal, O., and Ourednik, A.: Polygraphic study in the so-called Pickwickian syndrome. In Gastaut, H., Lugaresi, E., Berti Ceroni, G., and Coccagna, G. (Eds.), *The Abnormalities of Sleep in Man*. Bologna: Aulo Gaggi, 1968, pp. 223-229.

27. Burwell, C. S., Robin, E. D., Whaley, R. D., and Bickelmann, A. G.: Extreme obesity associated with alveolar hypoventilation—A Pickwickian syndrome. *Am. J. Med.,* 21:811-818, 1956.

28. Caldwell, D. F., and Domino, E. F.: Electroencephalographic and eye movement patterns during sleep in chronic schizophrenic patients. *Electroencephalogr. Clin. Neurophysiol.,* 22:414-420, 1967.

29. Cameron, W. B.: Some observations and a hypothesis concerning sleep-talking. *Psychiatry,* 15:95-96, 1952.

30. Castellotti, V., and Pittaluga, E.: Rilievi elettroencefalografici durante sonno spontaneo nell'epilessia "morfeica." *Riv. Neurol.,* 35: 568-587, 1965.

31. Chee, P. H. Y.: Ocular manifestations of narcolepsy. *Br. J. Ophthalmol.,* 52:54-56, 1968.

32. Child, C. M.: Statistics of "unconscious cerebration." *Am. J. Psychol.,* 5:453-463, 1892.

33. Coccagna, G., Petrella, A., Berti Ceroni, G., Lugaresi, E., and Pazzaglia, P.: Polygraphic contribution to hypersomnia and respiratory troubles in the Pickwickian syndrome. In Gastaut, H., Lugaresi, E., Berti Ceroni, G., and Coccagna, G. (Eds.), *The Abnormalities of Sleep in Man.* Bologna: Aulo Gaggi, 1968, pp. 215-221.

34. Cohen, H. D., Shapiro, A., Goodenough, D. R., and Saunders, D.: The EEG during stage 4 sleep-talking. Paper presented at the Annual Meeting of the Association for the Psychophysiological Study of Sleep, Washington, D. C., March, 1965.

35. Cohn, R., and Cruvant, B. A.: Relation of narcolepsy to the epilepsies. *Arch. Neurol. Psychiatry,* 51:163-170, 1944.

36. Crisp, A. H., Stonehill, E., and Fenton, G. W.: The relationship between sleep, nutrition and mood: A study of patients with anorexia nervosa. *Postgrad. Med. J.,* 47:207-213, 1971.

37. Critchley, M.: Periodic hypersomnia and megaphagia in adolescent males. *Brain,* 85:627-657, 1962.

38. Critchley, M., and Hoffman, H. L.: The syndrome of periodic somnolence and morbid hunger (Kleine-Levin syndrome). *Br. Med. J.,* 1:137-139, 1942.

39. Daly, D. D., and Yoss, R. E.: A family with narcolepsy. *Proc. Staff Meetings Mayo Clin.,* 34:313-320, 1959.

40. Daly, D. D., and Yoss, R. E.: Electroencephalogram in narcolepsy. *Electroencephalogr. Clin. Neurophysiol.,* 9:109-120, 1957.

41. Daniels, L. E.: Narcolepsy. *Medicine* (Baltimore), 13:1-122, 1934.

42. Dement, W.: Dream recall and eye movements during sleep in schizophrenics and normals. *J. Nerv. Ment. Dis.,* 122:263-269, 1955.

43. Dement, W.: The effect of dream deprivation. *Science,* 131:1705-1707, 1960.

44. Dement, W., and Kleitman, N.: The relation of eye movements dur-

ing sleep to dream activity: An objective method for the study of dreaming. *J. Exp. Psychol.,* 53:339-346, 1957.

45. Dement, W., Rechtschaffen, A., and Gulevich, G.: The nature of the narcoleptic sleep attack. *Neurology* (Minneap.), 16:18-33, 1966.
46. Diaz-Guerrero, R., Gottlieb, J. S., and Knott, J. R.: The sleep of patients with manic-depressive psychosis, depressive type. An electroencephalographic study. *Psychosom. Med.,* 8:399-404, 1946.
47. Ditman, K. S., and Blinn, K. A.: Sleep levels in enuresis. *Am. J. Psychiatry,* 111:913-920, 1955.
48. Douthwaite, A. H.: Proctalgia fugax. *Br. Med. J.,* 2:164-165, 1962.
49. Drachman, D. B., and Gumnit, R. J.: Periodic alteration of consciousness in the "Pickwickian" syndrome. *Arch. Neurol.,* 6:471-477, 1962.
50. Duffy, J. P., and Davison, K.: A female case of the Kleine-Levin syndrome. *Br. J. Psychiatry,* 114:77-84, 1968.
51. Dynes, J. B., and Finley, K. H.: The electroencephalograph as an aid in the study of narcolepsy. *Arch. Neurol. Psychiatry,* 46:598-612, 1941.
52. Earle, B. V.: Periodic hypersomnia and megaphagia. (The Kleine-Levin syndrome.) *Psychiatr. Q.,* 39:79-83, 1965.
53. Echeverria Muro, J.-L.: Consideraciones sobre patogenia y tratamiento del bruxismo. *Rev. Esp. Estomatologia,* 13:25-34, 1965.
54. Elian, M., and Bornstein, B.: The Kleine-Levin syndrome with intermittent abnormality in the EEG. *Electroencephalogr. Clin. Neurophysiol.,* 27:601-604, 1969.
55. Ethelberg, S.: Sleep-paralysis or postdormitial chalastic fits in cortical lesions of the frontal pole. *Acta Psychiatr. Neurol. Scand., Suppl.* 108:121-130, 1956.
56. Ethelberg, S.: Symptomatic "cataplexy" or chalastic fits in cortical lesion of the frontal lobe. *Brain,* 73:499-512, 1950.
57. Everett, H. C.: Sleep paralysis in medical students. *J. Nerv. Ment. Dis.,* 136:283-287, 1963.
58. Every, R. G.: The significance of extreme mandibular movements. *Lancet,* 2:37-39, 1960.
59. Every, R. G.: The teeth as weapons. Their influence on behaviour. *Lancet,* 1:685-688, 1965.
60. Fadell, E. J., Richman, A. D., Ward, W. W., and Hendon, J. R.: Fatty infiltration of respiratory muscles in the Pickwickian syndrome. *N. Engl. J. Med.,* 266:861-863, 1962.
61. Feinberg, I., Braun, M., Koresko, R. L., and Gottlieb, F.: Stage 4 sleep in schizophrenia. *Arch. Gen. Psychiatry,* 21:262-266, 1969.
62. Feinberg, I., Koresko, R. L., and Gottlieb, F.: Further observations on electrophysiological sleep patterns in schizophrenia. *Compr. Psychiatry,* 6:21-24, 1965.
63. Feinberg, I., Koresko, R. L., Gottlieb, F., and Wender, P. H.: Sleep

electroencephalographic and eye-movement patterns in schizophrenic patients. *Compr. Psychiatry,* 5:44-53, 1964.

64. Fisher, C.: Psychoanalytic implications of recent research on sleep and dreaming. Part I: Empirical findings. *J. Am. Psychoanal. Assoc.,* 13:197-270, 1965.

65. Fisher, C., Byrne, J., Edwards, A., and Kahn, E.: A psychophysiological study of nightmares. *J. Am. Psychoanal. Assoc.,* 18:747-782, 1970.

66. Ford, F. R.: The tired arm syndrome. A common condition manifest by nocturnal pain in the arm and numbness of the hand. *Bull. Johns Hopkins Hosp.,* 98:464-466, 1956.

67. Franks, A. S. T.: Masticatory muscle hyperactivity and temporomandibular joint dysfunction. *J. Prosthet. Dent.,* 15:1122-1131, 1965.

68. Frohman, B. S.: Occlusal neuroses. The application of psychotherapy to dental problems. *Psychoanal. Rev.,* 19:297-309, 1932.

69. Gallinek, A.: Syndrome of episodes of hypersomnia, bulimia, and abnormal mental states. *J.A.M.A.,* 154:1081-1083, 1954.

70. Gastaut, H., and Broughton, R.: A clinical and polygraphic study of episodic phenomena during sleep. *Recent Adv. Biol. Psychiatry,* 7:197-221, 1964.

71. Gastaut, H., and Roth, B.: A propos des manifestations électroencéphalographiques de 150 cas de narcolepsie avec ou sans cataplexie. *Rev. Neurol.* (Paris), 97:388-393, 1957.

72. Gastaut, H., Tassinari, C. A., and Duron, B.: Polygraphic study of the episodic diurnal and nocturnal (hypnic and respiratory) manifestations of the Pickwick syndrome. *Brain Res.,* 2:167-186, 1966.

73. Gélineau: De la narcolepsie. *Gazette des Hopitaux,* 53:626-628, 635-637, 1880.

74. Gerardy, W., Herberg, D., and Kuhn, H. M.: Vergleichende untersuchungen der lungenfunktion und des elektroencephalogramms bei zwei patienten mit Pickwickian syndrom. *Z. Klin. Med.,* 156:362-380, 1960.

75. Gibbs, E. L., and Gibbs, F. A.: Diagnostic and localizing value of electroencephalographic studies in sleep. *Res. Publ. Assoc. Res. Nerv. Ment. Dis.,* 26:366-376, 1947.

76. Gilbert, G. J.: Periodic hypersomnia and bulimia. The Kleine-Levin syndrome. *Neurology* (Minneap.), 14:844-850, 1964.

77. Gonzalez, F. M., Pabico, R. C., Brown, H. W., Maher, J. F., and Schreiner, G. E.: Further experience with the use of routine intermittent hemodialysis in chronic renal failure. *Trans. Am. Soc. Artif. Intern. Organs,* 9:11-17, 1963.

78. Goode, G. B.: Sleep paralysis. *Arch. Neurol.,* 6:228-234, 1962.

79. Goodwin, D. W., Freemon, F., Ianzito, B. M., and Othmer, E.: Alcohol and narcolepsy. *Br. J. Psychiatry,* 117:705-706, 1970.

80. Green, L. N., and Cracco, R. Q.: Kleine-Levin syndrome. A case with EEG evidence of periodic brain dysfunction. *Arch. Neurol., 22*: 166-175, 1970.

81. Green, W. J., and Stajduhar, P. P.: The effect of ECT on the sleep-dream cycle in a psychotic depression. *J. Nerv. Ment. Dis., 143*: 123-134, 1966.

82. Gresham, S. C., Agnew, H. W., Jr., and Williams, R. L.: The sleep of depressed patients. An EEG and eye movement study. *Arch. Gen. Psychiatry, 13*:503-507, 1965.

83. Gross, M. M., and Goodenough, D. R.: Sleep disturbances in the acute alcoholic psychoses. *Psychiatr. Res. Rep. Am. Psychiatr. Assoc., 24*:132-147, 1968.

84. Gross, M. M., Goodenough, D., Tobin, M., Halpert, E., Lepore, D., Perlstein, A., Sirota, M., Dibianco, J., Fuller, R., and Kishner, I.: Sleep disturbances and hallucinations in the acute alcoholic psychoses. *J. Nerv. Ment. Dis., 142*:493-514, 1966.

85. Gulevich, G. D., Dement, W. C., and Zarcone, V. P.: All-night sleep recordings of chronic schizophrenics in remission. *Compr. Psychiatry, 8*:141-149, 1967.

86. Hallgren, B.: Enuresis. A clinical and genetic study. *Acta. Psychiatr. Neurol. Scand., Suppl., 114*:1-159, 1957.

87. Hart, H. H.: Practical psychiatric problems in dentistry. *J. Dent. Med., 3*:83-94, 1948.

88. Hartmann, E.: Sleep and dream patterns in manic-depressive patients. Paper presented at the Annual Meeting of the Association for the Psychophysiological Study of Sleep, Gainesville, Florida, 1966.

89. Hartmann, E., Verdone, P., and Snyder, F.: Longitudinal studies of sleep and dreaming patterns in psychiatric patients. *J. Nerv. Ment. Dis., 142*:117-126, 1966.

90. Hawkins, D. R., and Mendels, J.: Sleep disturbance in depressive syndromes. *Am. J. Psychiatry, 123*:682-690, 1966.

91. Hawkins, D. R., Mendels, J., Scott, J., Bensch, G., and Teachey, W.: The psychophysiology of sleep in psychotic depression: A longitudinal study. *Psychosom. Med., 29*:329-344, 1967.

92. Heyck, H., and Hess, R.: Zur narkolepsiefrage, klinik und elektroenzephalogramm. *Fortschr. Neurol. Psychiatr., 22*:531-579, 1954.

93. Hishikawa, Y., and Kaneko, Z.: Electroencephalographic study on narcolepsy. *Electroencephalogr. Clin. Neurophysiol., 18*:249-259, 1965.

94. Hishikawa, Y., Sumitsuji, N., Matsumoto, K., and Kaneko, Z.: H-reflex and EMG of the mental and hyoid muscles during sleep, with special reference to narcolepsy. *Electroencephalogr. Clin. Neurophysiol., 18*:487-492, 1965.

95. Hodes, R., and Dement, W. C.: Depression of electrically induced

reflexes ("H-reflexes") in man during low voltage EEG "sleep." *Electroencephalogr. Clin. Neurophysiol.,* 17:617-629, 1964.

96. Jacobson, A., and Kales, A.: Somnambulism: All-night EEG and related studies. *Res. Publ. Assoc. Res. Nerv. Ment. Dis.,* 45:424-448, 1967.

97. Jacobson, A., Kales, A., Lehmann, D., and Hoedemaker, F. S.: Muscle tonus in human subjects during sleep and dreaming. *Exp. Neurol.,* 10:418-424, 1964.

98. Jelliffe, S. E.: Narcolepsy; Hypnolepsy; Pyknolepsy. *Med. J. Rec.,* 129:269, 1929. (Cited in Wagner, C. P.: Comment on the mechanism of narcolepsy. With case reports. *J. Nerv. Ment. Dis.,* 72:405-416, 1930.)

99. Jung, R., and Kuhlo, W.: Neurophysiological studies of abnormal night sleep and the Pickwickian syndrome. *Progr. Brain Res.,* 18: 140-159, 1965.

100. Kales, A., Beall, G. N., Bajor, G. F., Jacobson, A., and Kales, J. D.: Sleep studies in asthmatic adults: Relationship of attacks to sleep stage and time of night. *J. Allergy,* 41:164-173, 1968.

101. Kales, A., Heuser, G., Jacobson, A., Kales, J. D., Hanley, J., Zweizig, J. R., and Paulson, M. J.: All night sleep studies in hypothyroid patients, before and after treatment. *J. Clin. Endocrinol. Metab.,* 27:1593-1599, 1967.

102. Kales, A., Hoedemaker, F. S., Jacobson, A., and Lichtenstein, E. L.: Dream deprivation: An experimental reappraisal. *Nature* (Lond.), 204:1337-1338, 1964.

103. Kales, A., Kales, J. D., Sly, R. M., Scharf, M. B., Tan, T.-L., and Preston, T. A.: Sleep patterns of asthmatic children: All-night electroencephalographic studies. *J. Allergy,* 46:300-308, 1970.

104. Kales, A., Kales, J. D., Walter, R. D., Jacobson, A., and Paulson, M. J.: Recall studies in children. Paper presented at the Annual Meeting of the Association for the Psychophysiological Study of Sleep, Gainesville, Florida, 1966.

105. Kamiya, J.: Behavioral, subjective, and physiological aspects of drowsiness and sleep. In Fiske, D. W., and Maddi, S. R. (Eds.), *Functions of Varied Experience.* Homewood, Illinois: Dorsey Press, 1961, pp. 145-174.

106. Kanner, L.: *Child Psychiatry,* 4th ed. Springfield, Illinois: Charles C Thomas, 1972.

107. Karacan, I.: Insomnia: All nights are not the same. Paper presented at the Fifth World Congress of Psychiatry, Mexico City, November, 1971.

108. Karacan, I.: Painful nocturnal penile erections. *J.A.M.A.,* 215:1831, 1971.

109. Karacan, I., and Williams, R. L.: Insomnia: Old wine in a new bottle. *Psychiatr. Q.,* 45:1-15, 1971.

110. Karacan, I., Williams, R. L., Bose, J., Hursch, C. J., and Warson, S. R.: Insomnia in hemodialytic and kidney transplant patients. *Psychophysiology*, 9:137, 1972.

111. Karacan, I., Williams, R. L., Salis, P. J., and Hursch, C. J.: New approaches to the evaluation and treatment of insomnia (Preliminary results). *Psychosomatics*, 12:81-88, 1971.

112. Karacan, I., Williams, R. L., and Taylor, W. J.: Sleep characteristics of patients with angina pectoris. *Psychosomatics*, 10:280-284, 1969.

113. Kazamatsuri, H.: Electroencephalographic study of petit mal epilepsy during natural sleep. I. Studies on nocturnal sleep of epileptics. *Psychiatr. Neurol. Jap.*, 66:650-679, 1964.

114. Keefe, W. P., Yoss, R. E., Martens, T. G., and Daly, D. D.: Ocular manifestations of narcolepsy. *Am. J. Ophthalmol.*, 49:953-958, 1960.

115. Kerr, W. J., and Lagen, J. B.: The postural syndrome related to obesity leading to postural emphysema and cardiorespiratory failure. *Ann. Intern. Med.*, 10:569-595, 1936.

116. Kleine, W.: Periodische schlafsucht. *Monatsschr. Psychiatr. Neurol.*, 57:285-320, 1925.

117. Kleitman, N.: Patterns of dreaming. *Sci. Am.*, 203: November, 82-88, 1960.

118. Koresko, R. L., Snyder, F., and Feinberg, I.: "Dream time" in hallucinating and non-hallucinating schizophrenic patients. *Nature* (Lond.), 199:1118-1119, 1963.

119. Krabbe, E., and Magnussen, G.: On narcolepsy. I. Familial narcolepsy. *Acta Psychiatr. Neurol.*, 17:149-173, 1942.

120. Kuhlo, W.: Sleep attacks with apnea. In Gastaut, H., Lugaresi, E., Berti Ceroni, G., and Coccagna, G. (Eds.), *The Abnormalities of Sleep in Man*. Bologna: Aulo Gaggi, 1968, pp. 205-207.

121. Kupfer, D. J., Wyatt, R. J., Scott, J., and Snyder, F.: Sleep disturbance in acute schizophrenic patients. *Am. J. Psychiatry*, 126: 1213-1223, 1970.

122. Langworthy, O. R., and Betz, B. J.: Narcolepsy as a type of response to emotional conflicts. *Psychosom. Med.*, 6:211-226, 1944.

123. Laubscher, B. J. F.: Dissociation and somnambulism. *J. Med. Assoc. South Africa*, 5:12-14, 1931.

124. Laughlin, H. P.: The dissociation reactions. Dissociation, double personality, depersonalization, amnesia, fugue states, somnambulism, and hypnosis. *Med. Ann. D.C.*, 22:541-551, 578, 1953.

125a. Levin, M.: Narcolepsy (Gélineau's syndrome) and other varieties of morbid somnolence. *Arch. Neurol. Psychiatry*, 22:1172-1200, 1929.

125b. Levin, M.: Periodic somnolence and morbid hunger: A new syndrome. *Brain*, 59:494-504, 1936.

126. Lindner, R. M.: Hypnoanalysis in a case of hysterical somnambulism. *Psychoanal. Rev.*, 32:325-339, 1945.

127. Loewenfeld, L.: Ueber narkolepsie. *Munch. Med. Wochenschr.,* 49: 1041-1045, 1902.
128. Luby, E. D., and Caldwell, D. F.: Sleep deprivation and EEG slow wave activity in chronic schizophrenia. *Arch. Gen. Psychiatry,* 17: 361-364, 1967.
129. Lugaresi, E.: Brief clinical and physiopathogenetic remarks on narco-cataplexic syndromes. *Electroencephalogr. Clin. Neurophysiol.,* 13: 136, 1961.
130. Lugaresi, E., Coccagna, G., and Berti Ceroni, G.: Syndrome de Pick-wick et syndrome d'hypoventilation alvéolaire primaire. *Acta Neurol. Psychiatr. Belg.,* 68:15-25, 1968.
131. McCrary, J. A., and Smith, J. L.: Cortical dyschromatopsia in narco-lepsy. *Am. J. Ophthalmol.,* 64:153-155, 1967.
132. Mack, J. E.: *Nightmares and Human Conflict.* Boston: Little, Brown and Company, 1970.
133. Marie, and Pietkiewicz: La bruxomanie. *Rev. Stomatol.,* 14:107-116, 1907.
134. Marks, J.: The Marchiafava Micheli syndrome (Paroxysmal nocturnal haemoglobinuria). *Q. J. Med.,* 18:105-121, 1949.
135. Mayer-Gross, W., Slater, E., and Roth, M.: *Clinical Psychiatry.* London: Cassell & Co., Ltd., 1960.
136. Mendels, J.: *Concepts of Depression.* New York: Wiley, 1970.
137. Mendels, J., and Hawkins, D. R.: Electroencephalographic sleep studies in depression. *Sci. Psychoanal.,* 17:29-45, 1970.
138. Mendels, J., and Hawkins, D. R.: Sleep and depression. A controlled EEG study. *Arch. Gen. Psychiatry,* 16:334-354, 1967.
139. Mendels, J., and Hawkins, D. R.: Sleep and depression. A follow-up study. *Arch. Gen. Psychiatry,* 16:536-542, 1967.
140. Mendels, J., and Hawkins, D. R.: The psychophysiology of sleep in depression. *Ment. Hyg.,* 51:501-511, 1967.
141. Mitchell, S. A., Dement, W. C., and Gulevich, G. D.: The so-called "idiopathic" narcolepsy syndrome. Paper presented at the Annual Meeting of the Association for the Psychophysiological Study of Sleep, Gainesville, Florida, March, 1966.
142. Nadler, S. C.: Bruxism, a classification: Critical review. *J. Am. Dent. Assoc.,* 54:615-622, 1957.
143. Notkin, J., and Jelliffe, S. E.: The narcolepsies. Cryptogenic and symptomatic types. *Arch. Neurol. Psychiatry,* 31:615-634, 1934.
144. Nowlin, J. B., Troyer, W. G., Jr., Collins, W. S., Silverman, G., Nichols, C. R., McIntosh, H. D., Estes, E. H., Jr., and Bogdonoff, M. D.: The association of nocturnal angina pectoris with dreaming. *Ann. Intern. Med.,* 63:1040-1046, 1965.
145. Noyes, A. P., and Kolb, L. C.: *Modern Clinical Psychiatry.* Philadelphia: W. B. Saunders Company, 1958.
146. Onheiber, P., White, P. T., DeMyer, M. K., and Ottinger, D. R.:

Sleep and dream patterns of child schizophrenics. *Arch. Gen. Psychiatry*, 12:568-571, 1965.

147. Oswald, I.: Sleep and its disorders. In Vinken, P. J., and Bruyn, G. W. (Eds.), *Handbook of Clinical Neurology, Vol.* 3. Amsterdam: North-Holland Publishing Co., 1969, pp. 80-111.

148. Oswald, I.: *Sleeping and Waking. Physiology and Psychology.* Amsterdam: Elsevier, 1962.

149. Oswald, I., Berger, R. J., Jaramillo, R. A., Keddie, K. M. G., Olley, P. C., and Plunkett, G. B.: Melancholia and barbiturates: A controlled EEG, body and eye movement study of sleep. *Br. J. Psychiatry*, 109:66-78, 1963.

150. Passouant, P., Cadilhac, J., Baldy-Moulinier, M., and Mion, C.: Étude du sommeil nocturne chez des urémiques chroniques soumis à une épuration extrarénale. *Electroencephalogr. Clin. Neurophysiol.*, 29:441-449, 1970.

151. Passouant, P., Cadilhac, J., and Delange, M.: Indications apportées par l'étude du sommeil de nuit sur la physiopathologies des épilepsies. *Int. J. Neurol.*, 5:207-216, 1965.

152. Perlstein, M. A., and Barnett, H. E.: Nature and recognition of cerebral palsy in infancy. *J.A.M.A.*, 148:1389-1397, 1952.

153. Pierce, C. M., and Lipcon, H. H.: Somnambulism. Electroencephalographic studies and related findings. *U.S. Armed Forces Med. J.*, 7:1419-1426, 1956.

154. Pierce, C. M., Mathis, J. L., and Jabbour, J. T.: Dream patterns in narcoleptic and hydranencephalic patients. *Am. J. Psychiatry*, 122: 402-404, 1965.

155. Pierce, C. M., Whitman, R. M., Maas, J. W., and Gay, M. L.: Enuresis and dreaming. Experimental studies. *Arch. Gen. Psychiatry*, 4:166-170, 1961.

156. Pond, D. A.: Narcolepsy: A brief critical review and study of eight cases. *J. Ment. Sci.*, 98:595-604, 1952.

157. Radonic, M., Dimov-Butkovic, D., and Hajnsek, F.: The Pickwickian syndrome. *Lijec. Vjesn.*, 92:465-474, 1970.

158. Ramfjord, S. P.: Bruxism, a clinical and electromyographic study. *J. Am. Dent. Assoc.*, 62:21-44, 1961.

159. Rechtschaffen, A., and Dement, W. C.: Narcolepsy and hypersomnia. In Kales, A. (Ed.), *Sleep—Physiology and Pathology.* Philadelphia: Lippincott, 1969, pp. 119-130.

160. Rechtschaffen, A., Goodenough, D. R., and Shapiro, A.: Patterns of sleep talking. *Arch. Gen. Psychiatry*, 7:418-426, 1962.

161. Rechtschaffen, A., and Roth, B.: Nocturnal sleep of hypersomniacs. *Act. Nerv. Super.* (Praha), 11:229-233, 1969.

162. Rechtschaffen, A., Wolpert, E. A., Dement, W. C., Mitchell, S. A., and Fisher, C.: Nocturnal sleep of narcoleptics. *Electroencephalogr. Clin. Neurophysiol.*, 15:599-609, 1963.

163. Reding, G. R., Rubright, W. C., Rechtschaffen, A., and Daniels, R. S.:
     Sleep pattern of tooth-grinding: Its relationship to dreaming.
     Science, 145:725-726, 1964.
164. Reding, G. R., Rubright, W. C., and Zimmerman, S. O.: Incidence of
     bruxism. *J. Dent. Res.,* 45:1198-1204, 1966.
165. Reding, G. R., Zepelin, H., and Monroe, L. J.: Personality study of
     nocturnal teeth-grinders. *Percept. Mot. Skills,* 26:523-531, 1968.
166. Reding, G. R., Zepelin, H., Robinson, J. E., Jr., Zimmerman, S. O.,
     and Smith, V. H.: Nocturnal teeth-grinding: All-night psychophysi-
     ologic studies. *J. Dent. Res.,* 47:786-797, 1968.
167. Robin, E. D.: Some interrelations between sleep and disease. *Arch.
     Intern. Med.,* 102:669-675, 1958.
168. Robin, E. D., Whaley, R. D., Crump, C. H., and Travis, D. M.: The
     nature of the respiratory acidosis of sleep and of the respiratory
     alkalosis of hepatic coma. *J. Clin. Invest.,* 36:924, 1957.
169. Roth, B.: *Narkolepsie und Hypersomnie.* Berlin: Veb Verlag Volk
     und Gesundheit, 1962.
170. Roth, B., and Bruhova, S.: Dreams in narcolepsy, hypersomnia and
     dissociated sleep disorders. *Exp. Med. Surg.,* 27:187-209, 1969.
171. Roth, B., Bruhova, S., and Lehovsky, M.: On the problem of patho-
     physiological mechanisms of narcolepsy, hypersomnia and dissoci-
     ated sleep disturbances. In Gastaut, H., Lugaresi, E., Berti Ceroni,
     G., and Coccagna, G. (Eds.), *The Abnormalities of Sleep in Man.*
     Bologna: Aulo Gaggi, 1968, pp. 191-203.
172. Roth, B., Bruhova, S., and Lehovsky, M.: REM sleep and NREM
     sleep in narcolepsy and hypersomnia. *Electroencephalogr. Clin.
     Neurophysiol.,* 26:176-182, 1969.
173. Roth, B., Figar, S., and Simonova, O.: Respiration in narcolepsy and
     hypersomnia. *Electroencephalogr. Clin. Neurophysiol.,* 20:283, 1966.
174. Roth, N.: Some problems in narcolepsy: With a case report. *Bull. Men-
     ninger Clin.,* 10:160-170, 1946.
175. Sadger, J.: *Sleep Walking and Moon Walking. A Medico-Literary
     Study.* L. Brink, Translator. New York: Nervous and Mental Dis-
     ease Publishing Co., 1920.
176. Satoh, T., and Harada, Y.: Tooth-grinding during sleep as an arousal
     reaction. *Experientia,* 27:785-786, 1971.
177. Scherrer, M., and Hadorn, W.: Pickwick-syndrom. *Ergeb. Inn. Med.
     Kinderheilkd.,* 24:59-79, 1966.
178. Schneck, J. M.: Personality components in patients with sleep par-
     alysis. *Psychiatr. Q.,* 43:343-348, 1969.
179. Schreiner, G. E.: Mental and personality changes in the uremic syn-
     drome. *Med. Ann. D.C.,* 28:316-323, 362, 1959.
180. Schwartz, B. A., Seguy, M., and Escande, J.-P.: Corrélations E.E.G.,
     respiratoires, oculaires et myographiques dans le "syndrome pick-

wickien" et autres affections paraissant apparentées: Proposition d'une hypothese. *Rev. Neurol.* (Paris), 117:145-152, 1967.

181. Shapiro, S., and Shanon, J.: Bruxism as an emotional reactive disturbance. *Psychosomatics,* 6:427-430, 1965.

182. Sieker, H. O., Estes, E. H., Kelser, G. A., and McIntosh, H. D.: A cardiopulmonary syndrome associated with extreme obesity. *J. Clin. Invest.,* 34:916, 1955.

183. Sieker, H. O., Heyman, A., and Birchfield, R. I.: The effects of natural sleep and hypersomnolent states on respiratory function. *Ann. Intern. Med.,* 52:500-516, 1960.

184. Simpson, R. G.: Nocturnal disorders of medical interest. *Practitioner,* 202:259-268, 1969.

185. Skinner, B. F.: *Verbal Behavior.* New York: Appleton-Century-Crofts, 1957.

186. Snyder, F.: Electrographic studies of sleep in depression. In Kline, N. S., and Laska, E. (Eds.), *Computers and Electronic Devices in Psychiatry.* New York: Grune and Stratton, 1968, pp. 272-303.

187. Snyder, F.: Progress in the new biology of dreaming. *Am. J. Psychiatry,* 122:377-391, 1965.

188. Snyder, F.: Sleep disturbance in relation to acute psychosis. In Kales, A. (Ed.), *Sleep-Physiology and Pathology.* Philadelphia: Lippincott, 1969, pp. 170-182.

189. Snyder, F., Anderson, D., Bunney, W., Jr., Kupfer, D., Scott, J., and Wyatt, R.: Longitudinal variation in the sleep of severely depressed and acutely schizophrenic patients with changing clinical status. *Psychophysiology,* 5:235, 1968.

190. Sours, J. A.: Narcolepsy and other disturbances in the sleep-waking rhythm: A study of 115 cases with a review of the literature. *J. Nerv. Ment. Dis.,* 137:525-542, 1963.

191. Sours, J. A., Frumkin, P., and Indermill, R. R.: Somnambulism. Its clinical significance and dynamic meaning in late adolescence and adulthood. *Arch. Gen. Psychiatry,* 9:400-413, 1963.

192. Spitz, A.: Das klinische syndrom: Narkolepsie mit fettsucht und polyglobulie in seinen beziehungen zum morbus cushing. *Dtsch. Arch. Klin. Med.,* 181:286-304, 1937.

193. Stern, M., Fram, D. H., Wyatt, R., Grinspoon, L., and Tursky, B.: All-night sleep studies of acute schizophrenics. *Arch. Gen. Psychiatry,* 20:470-477, 1969.

194. Stoupel, M. N.: Étude électroencéphalographique de sept cas de narcolepsie-cataplexie. *Rev. Neurol.* (Paris), 83:563-570, 1950.

195. Szatmari, A., and Hache, I.: Narcolepsy—clinical, electrophysiological and biochemical appraisal. *Electroencephalogr. Clin. Neurophysiol.,* 14:586-587, 1962.

196. Takahaski, Y., and Jimbo, M.: Polygraphic study of narcoleptic syn-

drome, with special reference to hypnogogic hallucination and cataplexy. *Folia Psychiatr. Neurol. Jap., Suppl.* 7:343-347, 1964.

197. Tani, K., Yoshii, N., Yoshino, I., and Kobayashi, E.: Electroencephalographic study of parasomnia: Sleep-talking, enuresis and bruxism. *Physiol. Behav.,* 1:241-243, 1966.

198. Teplitz, Z.: The ego and motility in sleepwalking. *J. Am. Psychoanal. Assoc.,* 6:95-110, 1958.

199. Terzian, H.: Syndrome de Pickwick et narcolepsie. *Rev. Neurol.* (Paris), 115:184-188, 1966.

200. Thacore, V. R., Ahmed, M., and Oswald, I.: The EEG in a case of periodic hypersomnia. *Electroencephalogr. Clin. Neurophysiol.,* 27: 605-606, 1969.

201. Thaller, J. L., Rosen, G., and Saltzman, S.: Study of the relationship of frustration and anxiety to bruxism. *J. Periodontol.,* 38:193-197, 1967.

202. Trask, C. H., and Cree, E. M.: Oximeter studies on patients with chronic obstructive emphysema, awake and during sleep. *N. Engl. J. Med.,* 266:639-642, 1962.

203. Tuke, D. H.: *Sleep-Walking and Hypnotism.* London: Churchill, 1884.

204. Van der Heide, C., and Weinberg, J.: Sleep paralysis and combat fatigue. *Psychosom. Med.,* 7:330-334, 1945.

205. Vernallis, F. F.: Teeth-grinding: Some relationships to anxiety, hostility, and hyperactivity. *J. Clin. Psychol.,* 11:389-391, 1955.

206. Vincent, J.-D., Favarel-Garrigues, B., Bourgeois, M., and Dufy, B.: Sommeil de nuit du schizophrène en début d'évolution. Étude polygraphique par télémesure. *Ann. Med. Psychol.* (Paris), 2:227-236, 1968.

207. Vizioli, R., and Giancotti, A.: EEG findings in a case of narcolepsy. *Electroencephalogr. Clin. Neurophysiol.,* 6:307-309, 1954.

208. Vogel, G. W.: REM deprivation. III. Dreaming and psychosis. *Arch. Gen. Psychiatry,* 18:312-329, 1968.

209. Vogel, G.: Studies in psychophysiology of dreams. III. The dream of narcolepsy. *Arch. Gen. Psychiatry,* 3:421-428, 1960.

210. Vogel, G. W., and Traub, A. C.: REM deprivation. I. The effect on schizophrenic patients. *Arch. Gen. Psychiatry,* 18:287-300, 1968.

211. Wallis, H.: *Masked Epilepsy.* Edinburgh: Livingstone, 1956.

212. Walsh, J. P.: The psychogenesis of bruxism. *J. Periodontol.,* 36:417-420, 1965.

213. Werry, J. S., and Cohrssen, J.: Enuresis—an etiologic and therapeutic study. *J. Pediatr.,* 67:423-431, 1965.

214. Westphal, C.: Eigenthümliche mit einschlafen verbundene anfälle. *Arch. Psychiatr.,* 7:631-635, 1877.

215. White, P., Dyken, M., Grant, P., and Jackson, L.: Electroencephalographic abnormalities during sleep as related to the temporal distribution of seizures. *Epilepsia,* 3:167-174, 1962.

216. Yoss, R. E., and Daly, D. D.: Criteria for the diagnosis of the narcoleptic syndrome. *Proc. Staff Meetings Mayo Clin.,* 32:320-328, 1957.
217. Yoss, R. E., and Daly, D. D.: Narcolepsy. *Arch. Intern. Med.,* 106:168-171, 1960.
218. Zarcone, V., and Dement, W.: Sleep disturbances in schizophrenia. In Kales, A. (Ed.), *Sleep-Physiology and Pathology.* Philadelphia: Lippincott, 1969, pp. 192-199.
219. Zierler, K. L.: Diseases of muscle. In Thomson, R. H. S., and King, E. J. (Eds.), *Biochemical Disorders in Human Disease,* 2nd ed. New York: Academic Press, 1964, pp. 598-656.
220. Zung, W. W. K., Wilson, W. P., and Dodson, W. E.: Effect of depressive disorders on sleep EEG responses. *Arch. Gen. Psychiatry,* 10:439-445, 1964.

3.

Recent Advances in the Diagnosis and Treatment of Sleep Disorders

ANTHONY KALES, M.D.
JOYCE KALES, M.D.

NINE YEARS AGO, we founded our Sleep Research and Treatment Facility—a comprehensive program which includes 1) a Sleep Laboratory, 2) a Sleep Disorders Clinic, and 3) Educational Programs directed toward physician education and consultation to governmental agencies and private industry. The primary goal of the Sleep Research and Treatment Facility has been to obtain and disseminate information which would be of direct and practical value to the practicing physician in the overall management of patients with sleep disturbances. First, sleep disorders are evaluated in depth in the sleep laboratory and then these findings are applied to a larger number of patients in our sleep disorders clinic. Finally, the conclusions and recommendations from these studies are made available to the general physician to assist him in the diagnosis and treatment of sleep disorders.

We carried out a number of all-night EEG and clinical studies of primary sleep disturbances, such as somnambulism (sleepwalking) (1, 2), enuresis (bedwetting) (5), and insomnia (3, 4, 6, 7, 8). In addition, we studied a number of medical conditions, such as bronchial asthma (9, 10), duodenal ulcer (11), and hypothyroidism (12) to determine their effect on sleep as well as the effect of sleep on the particular condition. These studies have led in many cases to findings which have answered questions relating to the diagnosis and treatment of clinical conditions related to sleep.

IS SLEEPWALKING THE ACTING OUT OF A DREAM?

Despite the popular notion that sleepwalking is the acting out of a dream, sleep laboratory studies of somnambulists, involving primarily children, have shown that sleepwalking incidents occur exclusively out of NREM sleep (1, 13) (Figure 1). The sleepwalker functions at a very low level of awareness and critical skill, and is totally amnesic for the event upon awakening. The sleepwalking episodes in the laboratory lasted from 30 seconds to several minutes. Investigators were able to induce these episodes by lifting the subjects onto their feet during NREM sleep. All incidents, whether spontaneous or induced, characteristically began with a paroxysmal burst of high voltage, slow EEG activity.

Psychiatric disturbances were not found to be primary in the child somnambulists studied in the sleep laboratory. Our psychological testing did not demonstrate any severe psychopathology (2). There was a heterogeneity of personality patterns seen, with a spectrum of psychopathology from mild to severe.

The most immediate concern in treating the sleepwalker is protecting him from injury through prophylactic measures, such as locking doors and windows, having him sleep on the first floor if possible, and removing dangerous objects (3). Follow-up studies have indicated that most child som-

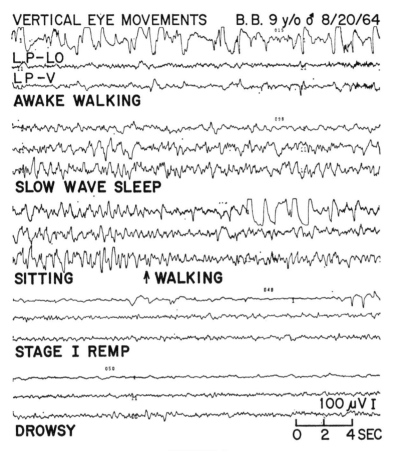

FIGURE 1

Comparison of the electroencephalogram of a sleepwalker at different times during the same recording session. The top recording was taken before the subject went to bed, while the third tracing was taken during a sleepwalking incident. The eye movements occurring during REM sleep are different from those recorded during the awake walk and sleepwalking (1).

TABLE I
VALIUM AND SLEEP STAGES
(Enuretic children)

		1	2	3	4
Baseline 3-4	21.6	3.9	46.8	11.7	16.1
Initial Drug 5-9	24.2	4.4	53.0	7.7	10.7
Home Drug 10-29					
Long Term Drug 30-31	25.6	3.4	62.0	7.9	1.2
Withdrawal 32-36	25.8	7.3	54.5	8.7	3.7
Withdrawal Followup 39	26.0	8.4	42.9	12.3	10.6

nambulists "outgrow" the disorder after several years, suggesting a delayed CNS maturation in these children (14). However, for cases where the sleepwalking is frequent and severe, as well as cases where the child does not "outgrow" the disorder, the use of stage 4 suppressant drugs is under investigation.

We have found that a number of drugs, primarily the benzodiazepines, such as diazepam (Valium) and flurazepam (Dalmane), very effectively suppress stages 3 and 4 sleep (3, 15-18) (Table 1). Use of these drugs with somnambulists in our laboratory has not resulted in a clear-cut decrease in the incidence of sleepwalking episodes. Dr. Charles Fisher has applied our findings with drugs that suppress stages 3 and 4 to patients afflicted with pavor nocturnus. These night terrors also occur exclusively out of stages 3 and 4 sleep, and he has found a marked decrease in the frequency of these attacks following the administration of Valium (19).

IS THE EFFECTIVENESS OF IMIPRAMINE (TOFRANIL) IN REDUCING ENURETIC FREQUENCY RELATED TO SLEEP STAGE ALTERATIONS?

Enuresis is the most frequent and distressing of childhood sleep disorders, and this situation is often aggravated by a lack of accurate information on the part of the parents of enuretic children. Sleep laboratory findings in great part contradicted the popular misconception that bedwetting represents hostile or dependent feelings on the part of the child. This is extremely important in preventing severe guilt and anxiety from being superimposed on the enuresis problem through parental mishandling of the bedwetting incidents. Very few bedwetting incidents occur when the child is awake. In addition, when the child is asleep the majority occur when dreaming is least likely, that is in NREM sleep, with some preponderance in the first third of the night (13, 20). Gastaut and Broughton (13) have also shown that if subjects remained wet following an enuretic episode and awakened in subsequent REM periods, they recalled fragments of dreams of being wet. This partially explains the misconception of a one-to-one relationship between enuresis and dreaming. Thus, when a child has an enuretic episode out of NREM sleep but his bed-clothing is not changed, he may subsequently incorporate the wetness into a REM period dream and in the morning actually believe that the enuresis occurred while he was dreaming.

In all cases of enuresis, particular concern should be directed toward counseling the parents. Parents of enuretic children invariably show deep concern over the disorder, and their actions often produce considerable guilt in the child. They should be educated as to the consequences of their reactions and informed that with patience and understanding, children generally outgrow the disorder.

In clinical sleep laboratory studies, we have evaluated the effects of an antidepressant drug, imipramine hydrochloride (Tofranil) in the treatment of enuretic children (5). Imipramine given twice daily in a total dose range of 75 to 125 mg markedly reduced the frequency of enuresis. This favorable clinical response is in agreement with previous clinical reports and is not related to any sleep stage alterations produced by the drug, but instead may be due to a peripheral action of the drug in increasing bladder capacity.

WHAT IS ONE POSSIBLE EXPLANATION FOR THE NOCTURNAL PAIN EXPERIENCED BY DUODENAL ULCER PATIENTS?

A common complaint of patients with duodenal ulcer is nocturnal epigastric pain and discomfort which awakens them and which may be relieved by milk or antacids. It had been previously established that these patients secrete 3 to 20 times as much gastric acid at night as do normal subjects (21). The question remained, however, whether this increase in nocturnal acid secretion was related to a specific sleep stage, or was a continuous process throughout the night. Studies in our laboratory with duodenal ulcer patients have shown that marked increases in gastric acid secretion usually occur during REM sleep (11) (Figures 2 and 3). Investigational studies are necessary to determine if REM suppressant drugs are of value in decreasing REM and gastric acid secretion peaks and if the benefits of such alterations outweigh the potentially detrimental aspects of REM rebound when the drug is withdrawn (3).

WHAT IS THE RELATIONSHIP OF NOCTURNAL ASTHMATIC ATTACKS TO SLEEP STAGES?

Patients with asthma frequently have attacks of dyspnea at night and complain of their inability to sleep well. We have conducted separate sleep laboratory studies with adult (9) and child (10) asthmatic patients. In the adult patients (9), the asthmatic incidents occurred throughout the night and were not related to any specific sleep stage. In the child patients (10), the asthmatic attacks were entirely confined

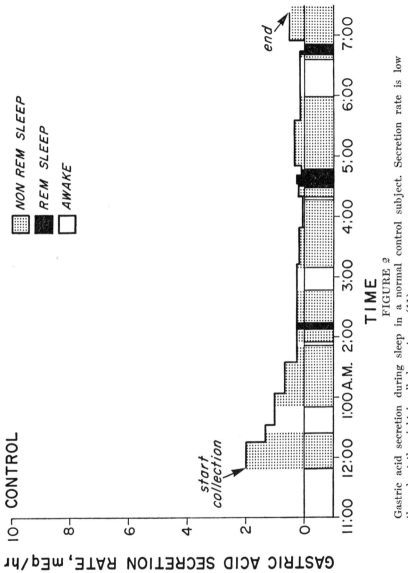

FIGURE 2

Gastric acid secretion during sleep in a normal control subject. Secretion rate is low throughout the night in all sleep stages (11)

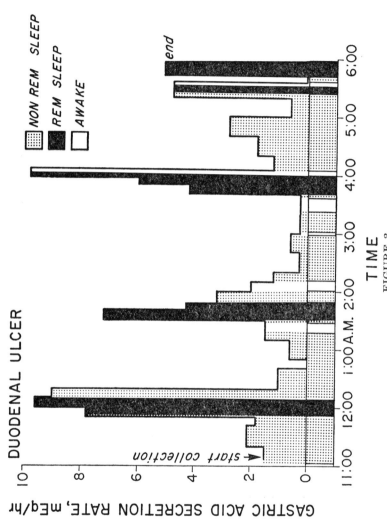

FIGURE 3

Gastric acid secretion during sleep in a patient with duodenal ulcer. Note the secretion peaks associated with REM periods and the subsequent decrease during NREM sleep (11).

to the last two-thirds of the night. While the total amount of stage 4 sleep was less in these children than in normal controls, no asthmatic incidents occurred in the first third of the night when stage 4 sleep predominated.

The results of these studies may have certain clinical implications. A significant increase in stage 4 sleep may be produced in normal subjects by moderate to vigorous exercise carried out at least several hours before bedtime (22). The lack of asthmatic attacks in children during stage 4 sleep, together with the finding that both adult and child asthmatic patients have significantly lower amounts of this sleep stage, suggest that exercise with its concomitant increase in stage 4 sleep may be associated with a decrease in nocturnal attacks (3, 10). Investigational studies are needed to evaluate this possibility.

INSOMNIA

While we have briefly discussed our sleep laboratory studies and findings in a number of clinical conditions, we would like to discuss in detail the total approach of our Sleep Research and Treatment Facility in the evaluation and treatment of the most prevalent sleep disorder—insomnia.

Through a combined approach of sleep laboratory and clinical studies, our Sleep Research and Treatment Facility has been increasingly involved in studies relating to both the evaluation and treatment of insomnia. These investigations have included both psychological evaluation of insomniac patients (4, 6) and sleep laboratory studies of the effects of drugs on sleep stages (15, 16, 23, 24), with the primary emphasis on determining the effectiveness of various sleep medications (17, 18). In addition, the effectiveness of psychotherapy or pharmacological treatment or combinations of both have been evaluated (4, 6).

This discussion of insomnia will also serve to illustrate how the Sleep Research and Treatment Facility, through its Sleep Laboratory, Sleep Disorders Clinic and Educational Programs, aids the physician in the diagnosis and treatment of sleep disorders.

EVALUATION

Psychological Testing

Minnesota Multiphasic Personality Inventories (MMPI) have been completed by 220 insomniac patients. Analysis of the first group of patients (N = 124) has shown a high degree of psychopathology in the group; 85% of the patients had one or more scales elevated to the pathological range (4). An elevated profile is defined as having at least one scale with a T-score of 70 or above.

The total insomniac sample is distinguished by 61% (N = 76) of the profiles having Scale 2 (D) with T-scores at or above 70, or in the pathological range. Scale 3 (Hy) had the next highest frequency, with 46% of the sample showing T-scores of 70 or over. This was followed by Scale 4 (Pd), Scale 7 (Pt), Scale 8 (Sc) and Scale 1 (Hs) having respective percentages of 45%, 42%, 39% and 31% with T-scores of 70 or above.

The most outstanding feature of this insomniac sample in terms of psychopathology was the high occurrence of depression. In addition to Scale 2 (D) being the single most frequently elevated scale in the 105 patients showing elevated profiles, it was among the three highest scales in 96% of these elevated profiles. Of the 76 elevated profiles, Scale 2 was the highest in 52% of the cases, the second highest in 32% of the cases, and the third highest in 12% of the cases.

Under 30 Years of Age

54% of the 48 patients in the youngest group had depression patterns (Scale 2 of (D) was one of their three highest scales). One pattern type accounted for 35% of the depression profiles in this age group. This was the "2-7-8" profile (Scales 2, 7, and 8 combined in any order as the three highest scales), which is characterized as an intellectualized, schizoid, ruminative depression and identity-disturbed profile. The remaining 65% of the depression patterns showed depression as part of a variety of other heterogeneous profile configurations.

Age 30-49

71% of the 48 patients in the middle age group had depression patterns. There were three pattern types which accounted for 57% of the depression patterns in this age group. 18% of these were "2-7-8" profiles (defined previously); 15% were "2-7-4" profiles (Scales 2, 4 and 7 combined in any order the three highest scales), which are associated with anxiety and depression in passive-dependent personalities; and 24% were "2-1-3" profiles, which are somatized depression configurations where health is a major preoccupation. The remaining 43% of the depression patterns consisted of profile configurations which can be loosely grouped into passive-aggressive depressions.

Age 50 and Older

82% of the 28 patients in the oldest age group obtained depression patterns. There was one major depression pattern in this group. 39% were clearly somatic depression patterns as defined by Scales 1, 2 and 3 (in any order) being the three highest scales. A broader classification of depression in this age group (which included Scales 1, 2 and 3 in any order and, in addition, profiles which had Scales 2 and 1 or Scales 2 and 3 as two of the three highest scales) accounted for 78% of the depression profiles. This broader group of somatized depression patterns is characterized by apprehensions and anxieties about health.

Thus, in this sample of insomniac patients, the depression in the younger age group appears to be qualitatively different from that in the older age group. Profiles in which Scales 2 and 3 are predominant, as in the older age group, predict a style of denial and repression. These patients focus on specific symptoms and difficulties and have many ways to cover over their depressions. Many seek to explain their depressions as caused by their depressive symptoms rather than vice versa, and their preoccupation with specific symptoms becomes a way to avoid facing the extent of their depressions. Thus, the MMPI results suggest that the younger patients, e.g., those with "2-6-8" codes, would more readily admit their depressions, anxieties, and self-doubts and be more willing to see their insomnia as related to their being depressed. The older patients, in contrast, test as prone to focus on their sleep symptoms so as to avoid facing their underlying if not more overt depressions.

Type of sleep problem (falling asleep, staying asleep, or early awakening) and use of drugs appeared to be much more strongly related to age than to type of psychopathology. Drug usage was strongly related to increasing age. In addition, there was a positive correlation among Scale 3, multiple sleep problems and drug usage, but the meaning of this with regard to psychopathology or age cannot be ascertained from our data.

Insomniac Patients (not using drugs)

The sleep of insomniac patients in the laboratory was compared to that of age-matched controls. As expected, the insomniacs had a significantly greater sleep latency and wake time after sleep onset (7, 8, 25). We have only occasionally found that a patient does not exhibit any insomnia in the laboratory after having reported a history of sleep difficulty. Thus, our results are not in agreement with those who report that many patients with clinical histories of insomnia do not manifest sleep difficulty in the sleep laboratory.

In comparing the insomniac patients and controls, there were no significant differences in the percentage and absolute amounts of REM sleep. Stages 3 and 4 sleep combined were decreased in the insomniacs but this was not statistically significant (7, 8, 25).

Insomniac Patients (chronically using drugs)

Patients who had been taking sleep medication chronically (months to years) were evaluated in the sleep laboratory under the conditions of their continuing to take their bedtime medication in the accustomed manner and dose (26). We found that despite large drug dosages, the patients experienced considerable difficulty in both falling and staying asleep, suggesting that with chronic use, these drugs are quite ineffective (26) (Figure 4). The effects on sleep stages of this chronic drug use are described below.

Insomniac Patients (before, during and after withdrawal of chronically used drugs)

Chronic use of multiple doses of hypnotic drugs was found to result in a marked decrease in REM sleep and a marked

NEMBUTAL

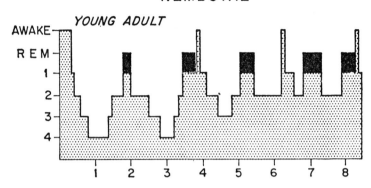

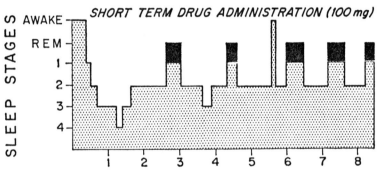

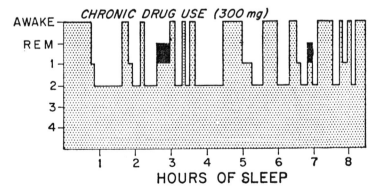

HOURS OF SLEEP

FIGURE 4

Sleep of a patient with chronic use of 300 mg. of Nembutal nightly. In spite of the large drug dose, it takes the patient almost an hour to fall asleep and there are twelve awakenings during the night.

decrease to complete absence of stages 3 and 4 (26) (Figure 4). During gradual withdrawal of the drugs, there was an immediate and marked increase in REM sleep associated with an increase in the frequency and intensity of dreaming (23, 24, 27-29) (Figure 5). Stages 3 and 4 slowly returned to baseline levels (i.e. for control subjects) without any rebound above baseline. With gradual withdrawal. the insomnia of the patients did not worsen and in some cases sleep improved.

Evaluation of Effectiveness of Drugs in Inducing and Maintaining Sleep

In our initial studies in the sleep laboratory, we were primarily interested in the effects of the drugs on sleep stages (15, 16, 23, 24) (Table 2). However, during the last several years we have extensively evaluated the effectiveness of hypnotic drugs in inducing and maintaining sleep, as well as the duration of this effectiveness (17, 18, 30, 31). The primary protocol used for evaluating this effectiveness is a 22-consecutive-night design utilizing insomniac subjects. The design is as follows, where P = placebo, D = drug, Lab = nights spent in the sleep laboratory, and Home = nights spent at home: 1-4, P, Lab; 5-7, D, Lab; 8-15, D, Home, 16-18, D, Lab; 19-22, P, Lab. The first placebo night allows for adaptation to the laboratory environment and then on nights 2-4 baseline measurements are obtained. On nights 5-7 initial and short-term drug effectiveness in inducing and maintaining sleep is measured, nights 17-18 mark the end of the two-week period of drug administration and these laboratory nights allow for determining if the drug is still effective or if tolerance has developed. Table 3 illustrates this 22-night protocol for evaluating the effectiveness of hypnotic drugs (17, 30).

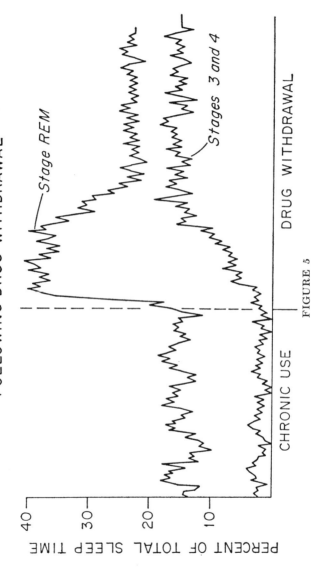

SLEEP PATTERNS DURING CHRONIC DRUG USE AND
FOLLOWING DRUG WITHDRAWAL

Stage REM

Stages 3 and 4

CHRONIC USE   DRUG WITHDRAWAL

PERCENT OF TOTAL SLEEP TIME

FIGURE 5

Following abrupt withdrawal of hypnotic drugs which have been taken for a
prolonged period of time, there is a marked increase in REM sleep with an
increase in the intensity and frequency of dreaming.

TABLE 2

STAGE REM ALTERATIONS FOLLOWING DRUG ADMINISTRATION AND WITHDRAWAL. EIGHT-NIGHT STUDIES

% Stage REM on Study Nights (Ni)

	Baseline Ni 3	Ni 4	Drug Ni 5	Ni 6	Withdrawal Ni 7	Ni 8	1st Drug Night	1st Withdrawal Night
GROUP A*								
Glutethimide (Doriden) 500 mg (N = 5)	27.0	14.3	16.2	18.0	31.4	30.7	−47.0	+16.3
Methyprylon (Noludar) 300 mg (N = 7)	25.3	18.4	18.9	25.3	31.5	31.6	−27.3	+24.5
Secobarbital (Seconal) 100 mg (N = 2)	20.2	15.3	19.8	19.0	21.1	21.2	−24.5	+4.5
Methaqualone (Quaalude) 300 mg (N = 5)	23.4	18.8	23.4	21.6	27.6	22.4	−19.7	+17.9
Pentobarbital (Nembutal) 100 mg (N = 4)	21.7	18.3	21.1	20.9	26.4	25.6	−15.7	+21.7
Diphenhydramine (Benadryl) 50 mg (N = 2)	20.8	17.6	15.6	15.2	26.7	20.1	−15.4	+28.4
Promethazine (Phenergan) 25 mg (N = 4)	18.3	18.5	23.0	17.3	33.3	26.2	+ 1.1	+82.0
GROUP B#								
Chloral hydrate (Noctec) 1000 mg (N = 5)	23.0	21.7	23.7	22.4	23.3	24.8	− 5.7	+ 1.3
Diazepam (Valium) 10 mg (N = 3)	20.1	19.2	20.1	18.8	20.1	20.7	− 4.5	0
Flurazepam (Dalmane) 30 mg (N = 8)	22.5	21.5	18.0	19.1	21.9	22.3	− 4.0	− 2.7
Chloral hydrate (Noctec) 500 mg (N = 10)	21.4	21.3	23.0	21.4	18.5	23.5	− 0.5	−13.6
Chlordiazepoxide (Librium) 50 mg (N = 4)	22.6	23.3	18.6	21.9	21.3	22.7	+ 3.1	− 4.9
Methaqualone (Quaalude) 150 mg (N = 5)	21.2	21.9	22.9	24.2	24.6	23.1	+ 3.3	+16.0

* Group A = drugs producing marked alterations in REM sleep with drug administration and withdrawal.
\# Group B = drugs producing no change or minimal change with drug administration and withdrawal.
N = number of subjects.

TABLE 3

22-NIGHT PROTOCOL FOR SLEEP LABORATORY—DRUG EVALUATION STUDIES

Night	P	D	Lab	Home	Reason
1	X		X		Adaptation to lab environment
2 to 4	X		X		Baseline measurements
5 to 7		X	X		Initial and short-term drug effects
8 to 15		X		X	Evaluation in home surroundings
16		X	X		Readaptation to laboratory
17 & 18		X	X		Long-term (2 wks) drug effectiveness
19 to 22	X		X		Evaluation of withdrawal effects

Throughout each study, whether they sleep at home or in the laboratory, subjects complete questionnaires each morning just after awakening. The subjects estimate the time it took them to fall asleep, number of awakenings, and soundness of sleep. These subjective reports are then compared with the actual EEG findings.

For this protocol, subjects are screened so that there is no history of significant medical illness or history of use of sleep medication or other psychoactive drugs, at least within the last several weeks. During the study, subjects are instructed to refrain from napping, to avoid use of any other drugs, including alcohol, and to maintain uniform daily levels of physical activity.

We have evaluated individually the following drugs and dosages with this 22-night protocol: chloral hydrate (Noc-

TABLE 4

DRUG EFFECTIVENESS
A COMPARISON OF FIVE HYPNOTIC AGENTS:
22-NIGHT SCHEDULE

CHLORAL HYDRATE (1000 MG.)

	Nights	Sleep Latency (minutes)	Wake Time (minutes)	Number of Wakes	Total Sleep %
Baseline	2-4	52.5	21.4	9.2	85.6
Drug	5-7	31.3	23.6	9.1	89.3
Drug	17-18	43.7	11.7	5.2	89.1
Withdrawal	19-22	61.2	8.8	5.7	86.2

METHAQUALONE (300 MG)

Baseline	2-4	39.9	76.2	10.8	75.8
Drug	5-7	26.1	47.5	5.2	84.7
Drug	17-8	27.8	80.5	7.5	77.4
Withdrawal	19-22	27.3	136.9	11.6	65.3

GLUTETHIMIDE (500 MG)

Baseline	2-4	76.2	13.7	6.8	82.7
Drug	5-7	38.0	19.7	10.0	88.7
Drug	17-18	90.2	16.4	6.6	79.1
Withdrawal	19-22	62.9	23.3	6.5	83.1

SECOBARBITAL (100 MG)

Baseline	2-4	29.3	57.7	11.6	81.9
Drug	5-7	17.6	20.7	8.4	92.0
Drug	17-18	30.0	47.0	6.6	84.0
Withdrawal	19-22	19.8	63.8	10.1	82.6

FLURAZEPAM (30 MG)

Baseline	2-4	35.8	14.3	4.1	90.0
Drug	5-7	13.9	5.0	2.7	96.4
Drug	17-18	21.2	3.8	2.3	94.7
Withdrawal	19-22	25.4	10.4	3.2	92.2

tec) 100 mg; flurazepam (Dalmane) 30 mg; glutethimide (Doriden) 500 mg; methaqualone (Sopor) 150 and 300 mg; and secobarbital (Seconal) 100 mg. We found that all of the drugs were intially moderately to markedly effective in inducing or maintaining sleep, or both (4, 17) (Table 4). However, we found that at the end of the two-week period of drug administration, decreased effectiveness had developed with all of these drugs except flurazepam. In the studies with chloral hydrate, glutethimide, methaqualone and seco-barbital, the subjective reports obtained each morning were essentially in agreement with the EEG findings. On the first set of drug nights, the patient felt that sleep induction or maintenance, or both, was improved; but as drug adminis-tration continued, the patients indicated a decrease in effec-tiveness for the drug, i.e., the development of tolerance.

Flurazepam administration resulted in a significant de-crease in sleep latency, wake time after sleep onset, and the total number of wakes (17) (Table 4). These favorable changes for both sleep induction and sleep maintenance were maintained throughout the two-week drug administra-tion period as evidenced by the subjective reports while at home (nights 8-15) and the results of the second set of laboratory nights (nights 16-18). Sleep latency, wake time after sleep onset, and total number of wakes were still de-creased below baseline levels on the withdrawal nights (nights 19-22); this indicates a carry-over effect of the drug. The subjective reports in the morning indicated improve-ment in sleep and were in agreement with the EEG findings.

In a subsequent, detailed study (18), we further evalu-ated the hypnotic effectiveness of flurazepam. In the two groups of subjects (Groups A and B) who received fluraze-pam, there was significant improvement in both sleep induc-tion and sleep maintenance (Table 5). The third group of subjects (Group C) was studied only under placebo or no

TABLE 5

Effects of Placebo and Flurazepam on Sleep Induction and Maintenance

Group	Nights	Condition	Sleep Latency (minutes)	Wake Time after Sleep Onset (minutes)	Total Wake Time (minutes)	No. of Wakes
A	2-4	O	29.9	35.2	65.1	12.7
	5-9	D	13.1	11.2	24.3	5.7
	10-14	P	18.7	31.5	50.2	10.8
	15-17	O	26.2	38.1	64.3	11.4
B	2-4	O	63.4	40.2	103.6	8.0
	5-9	P	69.3	38.3	107.6	6.3
	10-14	D	27.0	15.6	42.6	4.5
	15-17	O	32.2	24.9	57.1	5.8
C	2-4	O	46.9	21.3	68.2	7.8
	5-9	P	42.7	31.6	74.3	8.5
	10-14	P	37.7	33.2	70.9	8.9
	15-17	O	41.0	23.8	64.8	6.7

O = No medication administered; P = placebo administration; D = active drug (flurazepam 30 mg) administration.

treatment conditions. We found that placebo administration did not significantly increase or decrease either sleep induction or sleep maintenance nor significantly alter sleep stages (Table 5).

In another separate study (31), we evaluated the effectiveness of an over-the-counter sleep medication containing a combination of methapyrilene hydrochloride 25 mg and scopolamine HBr 25 mg. Because of laboratory scheduling difficulties, the drug was evaluated over an eight-night protocol consisting of the following consecutive nights, where P = placebo and D = drug: PPP DDD PP. Two placebo tablets or active medication were given each night. The results showed that in insomniac subjects with moderate to

TABLE 6

EFFECTS OF SOMINEX ON SLEEP INDUCTION AND MAINTENANCE MEAN VALUES, N = 5

Night	Condition	Sleep Latency	Wake Time After Sleep Onset	Total Wake Time	Total No. of Wakes
1	Placebo	54.8	12.0	66.8	6.2
2	Placebo	32.4	12.2	44.6	7.8
3	Placebo	42.4	20.8	63.2	6.6
4	Drug	42.4	13.2	55.6	7.0
5	Drug	55.8	22.6	78.4	9.0
6	Drug	84.4	13.2	97.6	6.6
7	Placebo	65.4	29.4	94.8	8.2
8	Placebo	43.4	26.6	70.0	9.4

severe insomnia, the drug produced essentially no favorable effect either in terms of sleep induction or sleep maintenance (Table 6).

In addition to evaluating the effectiveness of various hypnotic drugs, we are also evaluating the effectiveness of psychotropic drugs (tranquilizers and antidepressants) in facilitating sleep. We found that doxepin (Sinequan) 50 mg was effective in maintaining sleep and that diazepam (Valium) 10 mg was effective in inducing and maintaining sleep in insomniac subjects (4). We are now conducting sleep laboratory-drug evaluation studies to determine if doxepin is also effective in inducing sleep.

Psychiatric Treatment

In addition to initial psychiatric interviews with any new patients, we have seen many of these patients in ongoing psychodynamically oriented psychotherapy (4, 6). We have treated some of these patients from two to three years, enabling us to gain a better understanding of the psychodynamics of the insomniac patient. The most striking feature noted in interviews with these patients is a marked denial of psychological difficulties. As a consequence, these patients see physicians for years without being referred; they present such a negative approach to psychiatry that they frequently do not progress to starting therapy. If they do succeed in entering into ongoing psychotherapy, there is considerable resistance to the treatment itself. This takes the form of viewing the insomnia as the primary problem rather than one symptom of a more basic, underlying disturbance. This leads to considerable preoccupation and obsession on the part of the patient regarding the specifics of the sleep difficulty, type of drug used, drug dosage, etc. to the point where the psychotherapeutic session is dominated by these factors and it is impossible to explore any psychological parameters.

We have previously emphasized that insomniac patients strongly resist seeing their difficulty in psychological terms, and instead focus on the physical aspects. However, we have found that the majority of these patients should and can be treated with psychotherapy, especially if the therapist has an active and direct approach.

Insomniac patients in psychotherapy frequently emphasize certain physical or other problems which, upon analysis, appear to be of a minor nature. However, at the same time they very frequently neglect to mention, and in some cases due to repression are totally unaware of, problem areas in their lives which are indeed quite significant. Thus, it is very important for the psychotherapist to be more active with the insomniac patient in exploring possible problem areas. Questions regarding the insomnia *per se,* type of drug and dosage to be used, etc., should be confined to the end of the therapeutic hour so that psychotherapy does not become grossly contaminated with these questions.

We have been struck with the difficulty that insomniac

patients have in expressing and/or controlling their aggressive feelings. Frequently, this takes the form of completely unexpressed feelings of anger or hostility. In some situations patients are able to express or act out their anger, but do so in an uncontrolled fashion. Often this lack of control is substituted by a need on the part of the insomniac patient to control or manipulate his sleep medication contrary to the physician's recommendations, either in terms of varying the drugs or dosages used, or both. This needs to be interpreted to the patient in terms of the immediate psychological insight and also because pharmacological treatment is frequently rendered useless by this "jiggling and juggling" of medication (4, 6).

Pharmacological Treatment

As previously mentioned, a significant number of insomniac patients were noted to have depressive patterns on psychological testing. In many of these patients we combined antidepressant therapy (Tofranil) throughout the day with administration of Dalmane 15 or 30 mg at bedtime (3). We found that the use of Dalmane combined with Tofranil was no more effective than Dalmane alone. Because of the effectiveness noted in our laboratory studies with Sinequan in maintaining sleep, we are evaluating this drug further. We are trying to determine if the drug is also effective in inducing sleep (the patients in the original Sinequan study had little difficulty in falling asleep so that the drug's effectiveness in relation to this type of sleep difficulty could not be evaluated). Since the drug has antidepressant properties, we also want to determine if it is especially effective in those insomniac patients with significant levels of depression.

Based on the effectiveness demonstrated in the sleep laboratory, flurazepam is our drug of choice in all insomniac patients, whether they have a significant difficulty either in falling asleep or staying asleep or both (3, 4). For most patients, treatment is initiated with a 15 mg dose at bedtime. Our studies have shown that the drug is more effective on the second, third or fourth night of consecutive use than on the first night. The patient is informed of this so that he does not become discouraged, as often happens with insomniac patients, regardless of the treatment. In cases where 15 mg of flurazepam at bedtime does not appear to be improving sleep significantly after one week of therapy, the dosage is increased to 30 mg. In those cases where the patient presents a clear-cut history of a severe and chronic insomnia, treatment is initiated with a dosage of 30 mg of flurazepam at bedtime. We have noted that if mild insomniacs who do not weigh very much are given a dose of 30 mg nightly, there may be a significant carryover in terms of drowsiness the next day.

In cases of mild insomnia or insomnia secondary to situational disturbances, pharmacological therapy alone is most often sufficient. In more severe or chronic cases, best results are obtained with a combined approach of psychotherapy and pharmacological treatment (3, 4).

An important part of the overall pharmacological treatment of insomnia relates to the management of a problem which is not only severe but prevalent—hypnotic drug dependence.

Drug Withdrawal Insomnia and Hypnotic Drug Dependence

While it is true that considerable data have been amassed from modern sleep research laboratory studies, we do *not* know the specific significance of the presence or absence of a given sleep stage (30). For example, while it was previously thought that REM deprivation led to gross psychological changes (32), the current consensus is that these changes do not occur. Thus, at this time it would not be correct to state that REM sleep, stage 4 sleep, etc., are necessary (30).

We have found that most hypnotic drugs when used chronically in multiple doses are relatively ineffective. If this is so, why do patients continue to take these hypnotic drugs and be dependent on them? Our studies indicate that this is due to a condition which we call Drug Withdrawal Insomnia, which results from both psychological factors and physiological changes involved with drug withdrawal. When a patient abruptly withdraws from the regular and prolonged use of multiple doses of an hypnotic, he frequently first experiences marked insomnia, i.e., difficulty in falling asleep. This insomnia is due to psychological apprehension over his ability to get along without the drug and an abstinence syndrome of jitteriness and nervousness. In addition, once the patient gets to sleep, his sleep is frequently fragmented and disrupted. Sleep research has helped to explain this aspect of drug withdrawal insomnia. If the hypnotic which is withdrawn abruptly is a REM suppressant, and especially if the drug was used in high doses over prolonged periods, there is a marked increase or rebound in REM sleep associated with an increased intensity and frequency of dreaming (23, 24, 27-29). These altered sleep and dream patterns disturb sleep and contribute additionally to the drug withdrawal insomnia.

Our studies suggest that drug withdrawal nightmares secondary to increases in REM sleep could also occur on actual drug nights (24). As with nightmares following drug withdrawal, they would more likely occur in patients taking drugs for long periods of time. Nightmares during drug nights are probably rare but may occur when short-acting hypnotics are used and REM sleep increases late in the night as the drug wears off. In addition, nightmares may occur on drug nights when an individual sleeps for a protracted period (nine to ten hours) past the duration of action of the drug.

Along with the serious problem of drug dependency, altered sleep and dream patterns may play a role in accidental overdosage and attempted suicide (23). The occurrence of terrifying withdrawal nightmares in patients who are psychologically disturbed and who are sleeping alone at home may have tragic consequences. Most patients faced with this situation would assume that the unpleasant dreams and nightmares are due to intrinsic psychological factors. Under these circumstances, a patient may take a handful of sleeping pills to induce sleep and to obliterate the upsetting dream and, in effect, accidentally ingest an overdose. Other more disturbed patients may view their nightmares as an indication of increasing psychological deterioration and use the pills to attempt suicide.

Recommendations for Treatment

In treating drug dependency, the necessary measures are both curative and preventive. They include gradual drug withdrawal and, if necessary, gradual replacement with drugs that are effective in inducing and maintaining sleep (15, 23, 24). The results of our studies suggest that physicians should gradually decrease rather than abruptly terminate drug dosages during the withdrawal period. This is done when patients are dependent on large dosages of hypnotic compounds. Our studies indicate also that this withdrawal should be more gradual than previously suggested, i.e., withdraw one therapeutic dose every 5 days. Also, an individual taking only one or two capsules of a hypnotic nightly for more than several months should be treated in a similar fashion because of the underlying physiological alterations. The physician should also inform patients as to what may occur with drug administration and withdrawal. If a patient who has taken hypnotics for protracted periods wishes to withdraw from the drug, he should be told that he may experience clinical disturbances such as nightmares and insomnia as well as some agitation during the day, and that these changes are due to drug-induced physiological alterations rather than intrinsic psychological factors.

CONSULTATIVE AND EDUCATIONAL EFFORTS OF THE SLEEP RESEARCH AND TREATMENT FACILITY

Studies which produce meaningful results are not the only major responsibility of sleep laboratories specializing in clinical studies. The other crucial responsibility is through educative efforts to see that the results are properly understood and utilized outside of the sleep laboratory by the physician, general public, pharmaceutical companies and agencies such as the Food and Drug Administration (FDA). Since there are millions of insomniacs, it is impossible to study and/or treat even a small percentage of the total patient population in the sleep laboratory. However, the results obtained from the sleep laboratory and sleep disorders clinic now provide the physician with the means of more effectively evaluating and treating patients with disturbed sleep.

Figure 6 illustrates the total program of our Sleep Research and Treatment Facility. This consists of two major areas. The first, which we have discussed, includes the sleep laboratory and clinical investigations directed toward obtaining information on the diagnosis and treatment of disturbed sleep. Consultative and educational activities comprise the second area of the Sleep Research and Treatment Facility. The remainder of this paper describes these efforts to effectively disseminate the information obtained in the research studies.

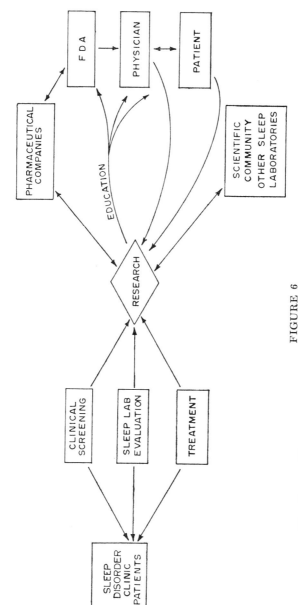

SLEEP RESEARCH & TREATMENT FACILITY

THE MILTON S. HERSHEY MEDICAL CENTER

THE PENNSYLVANIA STATE UNIVERSITY

FIGURE 6

The diagram illustrates how the Sleep Research and Treatment Facility, through its Sleep Laboratory, Sleep Disorders Clinic and Educational Programs, obtains and disseminates information on the diagnosis and treatment of sleep disorders.

Food and Drug Administration

Crucial to the value of any type of research protocol is whether results obtained from such a protocol have a significant degree of reproducibility from laboratory to laboratory. For example, we conducted several different investigations evaluating flurazepam 30 mg and found that the drug significantly improved sleep induction and sleep maintenance, produced little change in REM sleep with no rebound following drug withdrawal, and significantly decreased stage 4 sleep with a decrease being maintained over a short-term withdrawal period. Following our studies, four independent university sleep laboratory groups conducted separate evaluations of this drug and dosage (4). The results from each of these studies were in strong agreement with all of our findings, including those relating to sleep induction, sleep maintenance, REM sleep and stage 4 sleep, which demonstrates that there is a high degree of reproducibility of results obtained from one sleep laboratory to another (4).

Recently, a joint committee of the FDA and Pharmaceutical Manufacturers Association completed "Guidelines for the Evaluation of New Hypnotic Drugs" (33). One of us (A.K.) was fortunate to serve as a consultant on this committee. The new guidelines contain specific requirements for sleep laboratory evaluations of new hypnotic drugs. The protocols suggested take into consideration our previous recommendations for adaptation, readaptation, using consecutive nights of study, evaluating the withdrawal process and using periods of several weeks of drug administration so that the development of tolerance may be determined. The FDA guidelines also utilize the sleep laboratory-drug evaluation results by applying some of these findings to traditional clinical studies. The sleep laboratory finding that the sleep of one night is dependent on that of the previous night has led to the recommendation that only one drug condition should be studied within a given protocol unless there is a sufficient "washout period" allowed between drug conditions.

Pharmaceutical Firms

Advertisements in medical journals for hypnotic drugs provide the physician with practically no specific information on the effectiveness of the drug or the length of the effectiveness. References listed are frequently not published articles, but rather information listed as "on file" with the pharmaceutical firm. Generally, the advertisements contain broad statements to the effect that the specific drug produces "peaceful, sound and uninterrupted sleep." Our efforts have been twofold with this problem. First, we have encouraged many pharmaceutical firms to obtain objective sleep laboratory evaluations of the effectiveness of their drugs. Second, we have recommended that any advertisements for the drugs be scientifically rather than aesthetically oriented and provide the physician with detailed information as to the type and duration of the effectiveness of the drug. As a result of these efforts, a number of advertisements for hypnotic drugs have appeared which provide the physician with considerable scientific information.

Physician-Patient

We are hopeful that as physicians become more knowledgeable in the findings of modern sleep research, especially sleep laboratory-clinical studies, they will approach nocturnal disturbances with the same diligence that they direct to daytime disorders. Not only will the patients be directly benefited initially, but an indirect benefit will also result as the physician obtains additional clinical information on these disorders, which in turn can be shared with the sleep laboratory-clinician.

One of our major educative efforts in educating physicians on sleep was a scientific exhibit, Sleep Research in Modern Medicine (34), which described normal sleep and dream patterns and, in addition, findings from the sleep laboratory which related to the evaluation and treatment of disturbed sleep. Over a two-year period, this exhibit was shown at many scientific and medical conventions, including: Clinical Convention, American Medical Association; American Pharmaceutical Association; American Psychiatric Association; Annual Convention, American Medical Association; American Academy of General Practice; and Aerospace Medical Association.

We have now prepared a second scientific exhibit (35), The Evaluation and Treatment of Insomnia, which as implied deals in depth with this sleep disorder. This exhibit was recently shown at the Clinical Convention of the American Medical Association and will also be displayed at other scientific meetings in the future.

In this presentation, we have discussed how we approach the evaluation and treatment of sleep disorders in our Sleep Research and Treatment Facility. The studies in the sleep laboratory and the Sleep Disorder Clinic form the first major portion of this program (36). Of equal significance are the educative efforts directed toward disseminating the information obtained to the physician, patient, pharmaceutical firms and government agencies.

REFERENCES

1. Kales, A., et al.: Somnambulism: Psychophysiological correlates: I. All-Night EEG studies. Arch. Gen. Psychiat., 14:586-594, 1966.
2. Kales, A., et al.: Somnambulism: Psychophysiological correlates: II. Psychiatric interviews, psychological testing and discussion. Arch. Gen. Psychiat., 14:595-604, 1966.

3. Kales, A. and Kales, J. D.: Evaluation, diagnosis and treatment of clinical conditions related to sleep. *JAMA*, 213:2229-2234, 1970.
4. Kales, A. and Cary, G.: Treating insomnia. In: "Psychiatry—1971," *Medical World News Supplement* (E. Robins, Ed.): 55-56, 1971.
5. Kales, A., et al.: Sleep laboratory and clinical studies of the effects of Tofranil, Valium and placebo on sleep stages and enuresis. *Psychophysiol.*, 7:348, 1971.
6. Kales, A. and Cary, G.: Clinical implications of sleep." In: "Psychiatry —1970," *Medical World News Supplement* (E. Robins, Ed.): 62-63, 1970.
7. Kales, A., et al.: Sleep patterns of insomniac subjects: Further studies. *Psychophysiol.*, 9:137, 1972.
8. Kales, A. et al.: Electrophysiological and psychological studies of insomnia. *Psychophysiol.*, 6:255, 1969.
9. Kales, A., et al.: Sleep studies in asthmatic adults: Relationship of attacks to sleep stage and time of night. *J. Allerg.*, 41:164-173, 1968.
10. Kales, A., et al.: Sleep patterns of asthmatic children: All-Night EEG studies. *J. Allerg.*, 46:300-308, 1970.
11. Armstrong, R. H., et al.: Dreams and gastric secretions in duodenal ulcer patients. *New Physician*, 14:241-243, 1965.
12. Kales, A., et al.: All night sleep studies in hypothyroid patients, before and after treatment. *J. Clin. Endocrin.*, 27:1593-1599, 1967.
13. Gastaut, H. and Broughton, R. A.: A clinical and polygraphic study of episodic phenomena during sleep. *Recent Adv. Biol. Psychiat.*, 7:197-221, 1964.
14. Kales, A. and Jacobson, A.: Clinical and electrophysiological studies of somnambulism. In Critchley M. and Gastaut, H., *Abnormalities of Sleep in Man* (XVth European Meeting on Electroencephalography, Bologna, Italy), 1969, pp. 296-302.
15. Kales, A. (Ed.): Drug dependency, investigations of stimulants and depressants. UCLA Interdepartmental Conference. *Ann. Intern. Med.*, 70:591-614, 1970.
16. Kales, A., et al.: Hypnotics and altered sleep-dream patterns. II. All-Night EEG studies of Chloral Hydrate, Flurazepam, and Methaqualone. *Arch. Gen. Psychiat.*, 23:219-225, 1970.
17. Kales, A., et al.: Hypnotic drugs and their effectiveness. All-Night EEG studies of insomniac subjects. *Arch. Gen. Psychiat.*, 23:226-232, 1970.
18. Kales, K. D., et al.: Effects of placebo and Flurazepam on sleep patterns in insomniac subjects. *Clin. Pharmacol. Ther.*, 12:691-697, 1971.
19. Fisher, C., et al.: Effects of Valium on NREM night terrors. *Psychophysiol.*, 9:91, 1972.
20. Broughton, R. J.: Sleep disorders: Disorders of arousal?" *Science, 159*: 1070-1078, 1968.
21. Dragstedt, L. R.: Causes of peptic ulcer. *JAMA*, 169:203-209, 1959.

22. Baekeland, F. and Lasky, R.: Exercise and sleep patterns in college athletes. *Percept. Motor Skills, 23*:1203-1207, 1966.
23. Kales, A., *et al.*: Sleep disturbances following sedative use and withdrawal. In: Kales, A. (Ed.), *Sleep: Physiology and Pathology*. Philadelphia: J. P. Lippincott Co., 1969, pp. 331-343.
24. Kales, A., *et al.*: Hypnotics and altered sleep-dream patterns. I. All-Night EEG studies of Glutethimide, Methyprylon, and Pentobarbital. *Arch. Gen. Psychiat., 23*:211-218, 1970.
25. Kales, A.: Psychophysiological studies of insomnia. In: Heuser, G. (Ed.), *Clinical Neurophysiology: Diagnostic and Therapeutic Implications in Medicine. Ann. Intern. Med., 71*:625-629, 1969.
26. Kales, A., *et al.*: Effects of chronic hypnotic use. *Psychophysiol., 6*: 263, 1969.
27. Oswald, I. and Priest, R. G.: Five weeks to escape the sleeping pill habit. *Brit. Med. J., 2*:1093-1099, 1965.
28. Kales, A., *et al.*: Sleep patterns of a Pentobarbital addict: Before and after withdrawal. *Psychophysiol., 5*:208, 1968.
29. Kales, A., *et al.*: Sleep patterns during withdrawal of Tuinal: Effects of Dilantin administration. *Psychophysiol., 6*:262, 1969.
30. Kales, A. and Kales, J. D.: Sleep laboratory evaluation of psychoactive drugs. *Pharmacol. Physicians, 4*:1-6, 1970.
31. Kales, J. D., *et al.*: Are over-the-counter sleep medications effective? All-Night EEG studies. *Curr. Ther. Res., 13*:143-151, 1971.
32. Dement, W.: The effect of dream deprivation. *Science, 131*:1705, 1960.
33. Food and Drug Administration guidelines for the evaluation of new hypnotic drugs. Prepared by a joint committee of the Pharmaceutical Manufacturers Assn. and the Food and Drug Administration, 1971.
34. Kales, A.: Sleep research in modern medicine. Reprint from Scientific Exhibit shown at the annual meetings of: American Medical Association, American Pharmaceutical Association, American Psychiatric Association, American Academy of General Practice, Aerospace Medical Association, and American Neurological Association.
35. Kales, A.: Evaluation and treatment of insomnia: A. Introduction to sleep research in modern medicine and B. Sleep laboratory and clinical studies. Reprint from Scientific Exhibit shown at the American Medical Association annual convention, New Orleans, La., Nov. 29-Dec. 1, 1971.
36. Kales, A., *et al.*: Psychological evaluation and treatment studies of insomniac subjects. *Psychophysiol., 9*:91, 1972.